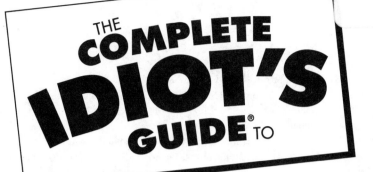

THE **COMPLETE IDIOT'S GUIDE**® TO

Knockout Workouts for Every Shape

Illustrated

by Patrick S. Hagerman, Ed.D.

ALPHA

A member of Penguin Group (USA) Inc.

ALPHA BOOKS

Published by the Penguin Group

Penguin Group (USA) Inc., 375 Hudson Street, New York, New York 10014, U.S.A.

Penguin Group (Canada), 10 Alcorn Avenue, Toronto, Ontario, Canada M4V 3B2 (a division of Pearson Penguin Canada Inc.)

Penguin Books Ltd., 80 Strand, London WC2R 0RL, England

Penguin Ireland, 25 St Stephen's Green, Dublin 2, Ireland (a division of Penguin Books Ltd.)

Penguin Group (Australia), 250 Camberwell Road, Camberwell, Victoria 3124, Australia (a division of Pearson Australia Group Pty. Ltd.)

Penguin Books India Pvt. Ltd., 11 Community Centre, Panchsheel Park, New Delhi—110 017, India

Penguin Group (NZ), cnr Airborne and Rosedale Roads, Albany, Auckland 1310, New Zealand (a division of Pearson New Zealand Ltd.)

Penguin Books (South Africa) (Pty.) Ltd., 24 Sturdee Avenue, Rosebank, Johannesburg 2196, South Africa

Penguin Books Ltd., Registered Offices: 80 Strand, London WC2R 0RL, England

International Standard Book Number: 1-59257-543-9
Library of Congress Catalog Card Number: 2006927521

08 07 06   8 7 6 5 4 3 2 1

Interpretation of the printing code: The rightmost number of the first series of numbers is the year of the book's printing; the rightmost number of the second series of numbers is the number of the book's printing. For example, a printing code of 06-1 shows that the first printing occurred in 2006.

Printed in the United States of America

Publisher: *Marie Butler-Knight*
Editorial Director: *Mike Sanders*
Managing Editor: *Billy Fields*
Acquisitions Editor: *Michele Wells*
Development Editor: *Lynn Northrup*
Production Editor: *Megan Douglass*
Copy Editor: *Krista Hansing*
Cartoonist: *Richard King*
Cover Designer: *Bill Thomas*
Book Designers: *Trina Wurst/Kurt Owens*
Indexer: *Angie Bess*
Layout: *Chad Dressler*
Proofreader: *Aaron Black*

Contents at a Glance

Contents

Introduction

Everyone has an image of themselves that's just a little different from what actually appears in the mirror. Whether it is an image of how you used to be, or an image of how you think you would look if you had someone else's body, we all seek a little adjustment here and there. Thankfully, you can accomplish just about anything you can imagine—with a little hard work and good old-fashioned exercise.

This is where a knockout workout comes in. The exercises you will find in this book are not another fad way of changing your body for a couple of weeks. This is a method of transforming your body into the look you've always wanted. There are no secret formulas, weird diets, or special exercises—just solid information that's based on solid science. A lot of these exercises are old favorites, and a few are pretty new. But it's not the exercise itself that makes the difference; it's how much exercise you do, how often you do it, and how much weight you use. It takes the right combination of exercises, sets, reps, and weight to get the results you want.

A knockout workout won't change your body overnight—that just isn't reasonable. It took you some time to get to the point where you are now, so give your body a few weeks to make a significant change. Then you'll notice your energy levels increasing and your clothes fitting better—and, all of the sudden, that image staring back at you from the mirror will look like a whole different person.

This book provides all the tools you need to set up your knockout workout, including resistance training, aerobic training, flexibility training, and nutrition. You'll come away from this book knowing exactly what you need to do to make it all happen. If you follow the advice and teachings here, you will be on your way to a fitter, more healthful lifestyle, and a body that everyone around you will envy.

How This Book Is Organized

The book is separated into three parts, each of which covers an essential component of your knockout workout plan:

Part 1, "Foundations for a Knockout Body," explains the basic principles of exercise, including the science of how much exercise is appropriate for you and your goals. It also explains how genetics and metabolism affect your body, and what you can do to manipulate them to your benefit.

Part 2, "The Well-Rounded Approach," pulls together the other three components of a complete exercise program: aerobic exercise, flexibility, and nutrition. In these chapters, you will learn how resistance training is complemented by a good diet that fuels your muscles, not your fat; how to stay loose and relaxed with a regular stretching program; and the importance of maintaining good cardiovascular health by working your heart muscle.

Part 3, "Putting Your Muscles to Work," is the heart of your knockout workout. These 10 chapters describe a variety of exercises for each part of your body. Each exercise is detailed in step-by-step instructions along with great illustrations showing you exactly how it's done. Additionally, each exercise has a few modifications included so you can adjust the exercise to your level of fitness.

Extras

Throughout the book, you'll find sidebars with quick and important pieces of information that summarize some of the text or add more information that's important to know. These sidebars include the following:

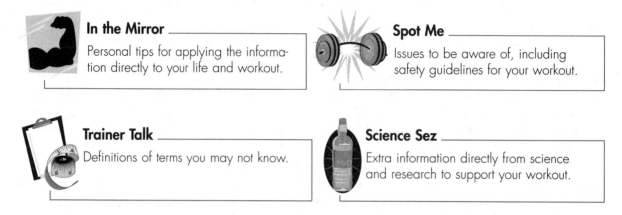

In the Mirror

Personal tips for applying the information directly to your life and workout.

Spot Me

Issues to be aware of, including safety guidelines for your workout.

Trainer Talk

Definitions of terms you may not know.

Science Sez

Extra information directly from science and research to support your workout.

So read up, start sweating, and good luck! The keys to success are consistency, commitment, and hard work—I know you can do it!

Acknowledgments

This is my fourth fitness book, and I still haven't run out of things to say or exercises to teach. Because there are so many people out there with different ideas of how they want to look, I decided that *Knockout Workouts* needed to be written. But I couldn't have done it by myself! I have to give the biggest thanks to my wife, Becki, who lets me sit in my office undisturbed while I'm writing and understands when I have that dreaded writer's block and need to procrastinate a while. She always offers just the perfect advice when I need it—she's amazing, and I love her.

To my friends and students who helped with the long days of taking pictures, a big thanks to Aaron Edwards, Michael Coday, Linda Farris, Pamela Geiger, Floyd Geiger, Rita Howell, Brandy Price, Lakeissha Sanders, Al Sorensen, Jocelyn Stroud, and Ron Walker.

Finally, to all my colleagues in the fitness industry: Many of you have helped me learn with your writings and teachings. Others have debated points with me to the end that we both come away with more knowledge. To those who have provided input on how exercise has affected their lives, thanks for intriguing my brain—and keep it up!

Trademarks

All terms mentioned in this book that are known to be or are suspected of being trademarks or service marks have been appropriately capitalized. Alpha Books and Penguin Group (USA) Inc. cannot attest to the accuracy of this information. Use of a term in this book should not be regarded as affecting the validity of any trademark or service mark.

In This Part

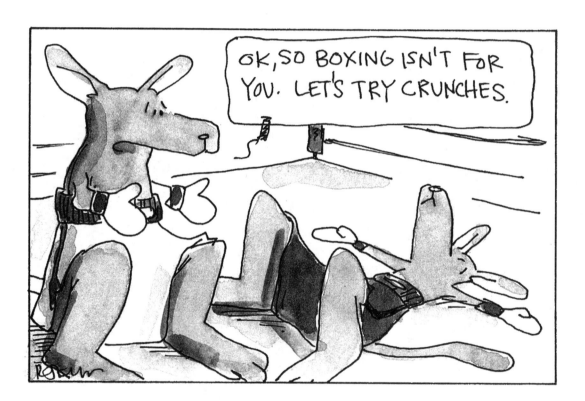

Foundations for a Knockout Body

Your body is a lot like an automobile. If you take care of it, keep it from getting wrecked, and give it plenty of good fuel, it will last a long time and take you all kinds of places. Unfortunately, most people know more about taking care of their car than they do about taking care of their body. The first part of this book teaches you all you need to know about keeping your body in shape, including why workouts are important, the ways your body will respond to exercise, and how to design a workout routine that will give you the knockout look you want. Chapters 1–4 are basically "everything you ever wanted to know about exercise but just never asked." I take all the confusion and hype out of exercise and leave you with the basic foundations of how to build a program that will put you on the road to changing your body forever. I'm sure you've heard this sort of claim before, but after you read this, you'll understand why I can say it with a straight face—it's no lie. This is so easy when you know where you are starting from and where you want to go. It's just like finding your way down the road with a great map—a piece of cake (low-fat, that is).

In This Chapter

- ◆ How do you want to look?
- ◆ Getting your exercise prescription
- ◆ Tailor an exercise program to your goals and your body
- ◆ Getting fit at any age
- ◆ Workouts wherever you go

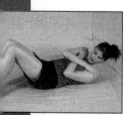 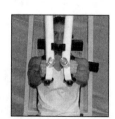 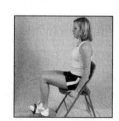 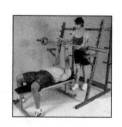 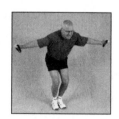 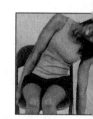

Chapter 1

Just What Is a Knockout Workout?

It happens every morning. You wake up, get out of bed, pry open your eyes, get dressed, and get ready for the day's events. But before you leave the house, I'll bet there is one more thing you always do—look in the mirror. Why do you do this? Simple—you want to know how you look and, more important, how other people will see you.

We all want to be seen looking our best, which often means having a great shape that we're happy with. When you look in the mirror, do you see what you want to see or something you would like to change? I'm guessing that since you are reading this book, you're searching for the perfect workout plan that will magically transform your body into an image you want to see in the mirror every day—an image that will lead other people to call you a "knockout."

Well, you're about to learn the key to a knockout body within these pages. This isn't a secret recipe or magical workout plan; it's just a simple matter of figuring out how you want your body to change and then applying the exercises that will get you that result. Before long, you'll have to tear yourself away from that mirror because the view will be fantastic!

We Aren't Talking About Boxing

What do you think about when you hear the word *knockout?* Does your mind lean toward the end result of two guys standing in a ring hitting each other in a contest civilized people call boxing? According to that Webster guy who knows the definition of every word, knockout means something along the lines of "sensationally striking, appealing, or attractive." That doesn't sound like a boxing match to me. It sounds like the way I want people to describe how I look. Don't you think so, too?

Of course, we all have our own personal definition of what constitutes striking, appealing, or attractive. The popular media would have you believe that supermodels are the essence of what we should all strive to look like. What makes models "super" anyway? Can they leap tall buildings in a single bound? The only time I've ever seen a supermodel is on television, but I see lots of people with great shapes every day. Some of them I'd even call knockouts.

There is no one definition of what a knockout is—just as long as it makes you go, "Wow, look at that. I look pretty darned good, if I do say so myself." In fact, I think I will say it, "Hey, you in the mirror there—you look pretty darned good. You're a real knockout!" My point is, what looks good is all in the eye of the beholder. We all have an idea of what we want to look like, so there is no reason we can't all describe that as a "knockout body."

Science Sez

Looking good isn't the only benefit of exercise; you'll also feel better! A knockout workout releases hormones known as endorphins from the brain, which cause feelings of happiness, contentment, and make every day seem better.

Now, to get this to happen, you're going to need a knockout workout. That's a workout that changes the body you have now into the body you want to see every day. As I said earlier, it's no secret, no matter what those infomercial people tell you. A knockout workout is all about putting the right pieces of the exercise puzzle together to make the vision in the mirror a work of art. So keep on reading because I'm going to teach you how to do just that.

A Prescription for Exercise

One of the first things you need to understand is that obtaining that knockout body is going to take different amounts of work for different people. If you get sick and go to the doctor, you wouldn't expect to be given the same medicine as everybody else visiting the doctor that day. We all have different needs based on our different bodies. Exercise doesn't come in just one form; each prescription is a little different and should be tailored to your individual needs and goals.

Science Sez

Exercise physiologists shorten the term "exercise prescription" to "Ex Rx," borrowing a little bit from the medical profession. By the end of this book, you will have devised your own Ex Rx.

Your exercise prescription is designed by choosing the exercises that fit your body type, your goals, your abilities, and how much time and effort you can put into a regular workout. We cover the specifics of which exercises to choose, how many you should do, how much weight to use, and when you get to rest in later chapters. What you need to know right now is that the plan you design from this book will be different from the one your best friend designs, or the plan for your mom, or your kids, or your uncle's best friend's cousin's next-door-neighbor. This is an individual approach.

The plans you see in magazines or on TV that are supposed to be the "10 best exercises to tone and firm your entire body in 8 short weeks"—or, my favorite, the "secret workouts of the stars"—aren't found in these pages. Why not? Because they don't really work! If they did, everyone in the world would already look fabulous, and you wouldn't be reading this book. I'm not going to say that the exercise program you put together here is the end-all-be-all of exercise programs—but it's going to be something that is designed just for you, with your particular goals in mind. This is not some cookie-cutter plan that everyone else is trying and failing with.

I'm just going to lay it all out there in plain simple language without trying to confuse you with a bunch of scientific jargon. You should understand that the science behind how the body responds to exercise (technically known as exercise physiology) is always changing as we learn more about the body and how to make it change the way we want to. You'll have the most up-to-date information available, and you'll understand how it all works so you can explain it to your friends, who will soon be envious of what you have accomplished.

Getting Fit Has to Fit

One of the neatest things about exercise is that anyone can do it—and I mean anyone! My favorite excuse I've ever heard for not exercising is, "I'm not in good enough shape to exercise." Isn't that absolutely ridiculous? How do you get in shape to exercise without exercising? It used to be a rule (and I use the word *rule* very loosely here) that exercise was only for adults, but not older adults. This type of outdated thinking was based on the idea that kids shouldn't exercise because it would stunt their growth, and that older adults shouldn't exercise because they're

getting too frail to subject their bodies to that kind of stress.

Thank goodness we now understand that none of this is true (look back and you'll see that I said it was based on an "idea," not any solid evidence). Science has shown without any doubt that exercise is good for everyone, no matter what their age, physical condition, height, weight, or favorite flavor of ice cream. In fact, exercise is fast becoming the first recommendation of medical doctors to help treat most of the chronic diseases that cause premature death.

In the Mirror
Exercise is recommended for everyone. Exercise programs can be designed for children as young as 2 to 3 years old and for adults over 100, for people with cancer and asthma, for women who are pregnant, and for those who just had back surgery—but they aren't all the same. You have to find a program that's right for your body.

Are you getting excited now? I hope so—I've just taken away any excuse you might have had to skip that next workout. It's time to get moving! But before you go skipping out the door and into the gym, you need to understand that not every exercise is made for every person. For any given exercise, there is a specific result attached. That result is directly tied to how you do an exercise, what muscles are involved in that exercise, how hard you work on that exercise, and whether you do the exercise correctly.

When you see someone doing an exercise and it looks like he or she is getting some good results from it, you have to take a step back and look at everything this person is doing in the workout. No one exercise is responsible for a person's entire look; no magic exercise can transform your entire body. Each exercise works certain parts of your body and certain muscles in certain ways. It takes a combination of several exercises to work your entire body. That being said, you can't just pick any group of exercises and have at it. You have to pick the exercises that fit you.

If you have a particular fondness for the bench press, that's fine—but is that bench press the best exercise for you? Maybe some other form of chest exercise would produce a better result for your body. I've found quite often that the exercises that do us the most good are often the ones we don't do for some reason. It could be as simple as the fact that you didn't know about that exercise, or it could be that you don't like that exercise. It's okay not to like an exercise. When this happens, you just move on to the next best exercise.

Above all else, your knockout workout has to fit your goals and your body. Each of the exercises you'll see in Part 3 of this book describe modifications that will help you find the best way to fit that exercise into your overall plan. I told you this was an individualized process.

Age Doesn't Matter

A long time ago, I started working with older adults who were living in retirement homes and nursing centers. At first I found that the "exercises" they were being instructed to do had very little effect on their body. Imagine catching a beach ball and tossing it to someone three or four times, and calling that an exercise session.

When I started challenging them to do things they had to work on, their bodies started getting stronger. Their muscles started regaining shape, and they started standing up straighter, looking healthier, and being able to get involved in activities that they loved to do, such as dancing and bowling.

Science Sez _____

Research has shown that a proper exercise program can produce increases in strength in older adults to the same degree that it does in young adults. Older adults might not lift the same amount of weight, but if you go from lifting 10 pounds to 20 pounds, that's a 100 percent improvement.

On the other end of the spectrum, it was recently believed that children shouldn't exercise before going through puberty because exercise would stunt their growth or cause injuries. At the same time, involvement in Little League baseball, football, and soccer reached all-time highs. Isn't that exercise? When enough data was collected, the fitness industry discovered that there never has been an indication of growth being stunted, and that children are more likely to get injured playing sports than during a supervised workout (something like 95 out of 100 injuries happen during sports).

The bottom line is that if you are old enough to be alive, you are old enough (or young enough) for a knockout workout and a knockout body.

Spot Me _____

No matter what your age or physical shape, you should make an appointment with your doctor to get a general physical before beginning any new exercise program.

At Home or on the Road

My wife travels for work all the time. She has to drive, fly, stay in hotels that don't have fitness centers, and eat in restaurants that may not have the healthiest food—but she keeps in shape. Having a knockout workout doesn't mean you have to join a gym or buy a huge exercise machine for your house. Plenty of exercises can be done with little or no equipment. Back in the days of the earliest Olympics in Greece, there was no local health club to go to with nice shiny barbells and an aerobics program. The people used what they had, which was usually just their bodies and some heavy rocks.

I don't suggest that you start lifting boulders, but you can always use the one form of resistance you can never get away from—gravity. The weight of our bodies is usually plenty to get a good workout when you can't make it to your gym. I haven't been to a gym to work out in years. Just a few pieces of small equipment, such as resistance tubing and stability balls (we talk more about home equipment in Chapter 3) are all you need to get a good workout. So no more complaining because you can't get to the gym—these knockout workouts can follow you anywhere.

The Least You Need to Know

◆ The goal of your knockout workout will be different from anyone else's workout because you are starting from a different point and have a different idea of what a "knockout" is.

◆ The time and effort you put into your program will determine what you get out of it. The harder you work, the better the results.

◆ Age has nothing to do with exercise. No matter how young or not-so-young you may be, a knockout workout can change your body.

◆ Gravity is a form of resistance we have to fight all the time so it's perfect for workouts on the road.

In This Chapter

- ◆ Apples vs. pears
- ◆ The body you're born with
- ◆ Building your metabolism
- ◆ Fat and muscle: not the same thing
- ◆ Bigger, but not bulging

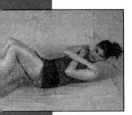 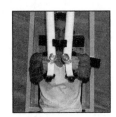 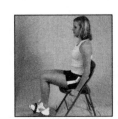 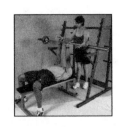 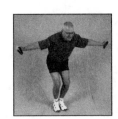 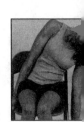

Different Strokes for Different Folks

Here's a news flash: everyone is a little different from you. We all have the same basic structure, but the look is always different. Yeah, I know that probably isn't breaking news—but think of it this way: if you tell people you drive a car, that really doesn't tell them much. If you say you drive a Ford Mustang, now they know that you like to drive fast. We are all human, but every human is a little different from the human next to them (even identical twins can turn out different). Each of us has a different idea of what constitutes a knockout body. What you have in mind for your body is probably different from what anyone else thinks. If you take a walk through your local mall, you'll notice that rarely are any two bodies shaped the same. If we don't all begin at the same place, it makes sense that your knockout workouts won't all be the same.

Your starting point is the genetics you inherited from your parents. Science has yet to find a way for us to easily change our genetics, but we can manipulate their results in certain ways to change your body's shape. This chapter is designed to enlighten you about how your body shape is determined, what changes you can make, and the different types of knockout workouts that will result in a whole new you. (But you'll still be human—I can't make you into a giraffe or anything.)

What's Your Body Type?

Exercise science textbooks usually mention three basic "body types": mesomorph, ectomorph, and endomorph. Because you probably don't read exercise science textbooks, let's just call them the skinny, fat, and muscular body types. I'll bet you've just classified yourself into one of these categories in your head. That's what I thought. So would you agree that every person on the planet is either skinny, fat, or muscular? How about tall or short? Big hands or big feet? Long hair or short hair? We could go on and on trying to place people into categories, but it just doesn't work. Not everybody is exactly skinny, fat, or muscular—they're probably somewhere in the middle of these three extremes.

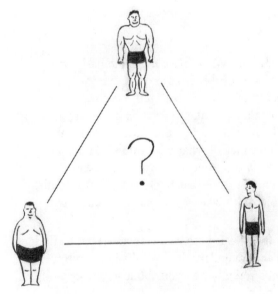

You probably fit somewhere in the middle of these three body type extremes.

Maybe you've heard of the "pear" shape or the "apple" shape. These refer to a person who carries more weight above the waist (the apple), and someone who carries more weight

below the waist (the pear). So can everyone be either a pear or an apple? I doubt it. I've seen bananas, cantaloupes, and even a peanut or two. In fact, the pear and apple characteristics are used most often to describe a person's tendency toward having heart disease. Those who carry more weight up top (the apples) have a higher incidence of heart-related diseases than the pears. Why? Part of it is because the heart has to work harder when there is more mass and effort located closer to it (around your chest). But we could describe the muscular guy as an apple shape. Does this mean that being muscular will cause you to have heart problems? No, it doesn't. The apple and pear shapes are concerned with fat mass, not muscle. If you are an apple because of extra fat, you might have a problem—but muscle is fine.

Science Sez

Research has shown that there is a correlation between heart disease and extra fat above the waist. Overweight people with an "apple" shape are at greater risk for heart attacks, coronary artery disease, and congestive heart failure.

So now are you totally confused about what shape you really are? Good. Because it really doesn't matter that much—you are about to change everything and reshape your body into a new knockout look! I just wanted you to be aware of the categories that a lot of people try to define us by. That really doesn't apply to you because very few of us fit the strict definitions of each category. A knockout look can be built from any body shape; you just have to focus on the areas of your body that need the most work and, at the same time, improve your strong points even more.

Changing Your Genetics

I'll start by saying that if I could change your genetics to make your body more beautiful, I'd probably be sitting on a beach somewhere writing this book instead of in my stuffy little office. Whoever figures out how to change a person's genetics will be the richest person in the world. So it goes without saying that it hasn't been done yet—no matter what those infomercials say!

We are each born with whatever our parents gave us, but this doesn't mean we'll end up looking like them. We can't change our genetics, but we can influence how our body responds to them. For instance, the worst-case scenario is that both of your parents were obese and had high cholesterol, heart disease, and all kinds of health problems. Will this happen to you, too? It could if you let it. But I'm guessing that because you have read this far, you want to change something about your body. If these are your parents, fear not. You can still be a lean, mean, healthy knockout machine.

In the Mirror

Facial features are about the only part of your body that you inherited from your parents that you can't change with exercise and proper nutrition. Your body's shape depends on what you choose to make of it.

Your genetics don't define how your body will look all by themselves. Exercise, nutrition, and lifestyle have a lot to do with it also. Imagine a set of twins, with one completely sedentary his whole life, and the other a fitness nut. They would never look like twins. What you do with the genes you're given determines more how you will look than how your parents look. The excuse "I have bad genes; I can't get

in shape" is the worst excuse I have ever heard (and I've heard it a lot)! You decide what you want your body to look like; then you plan your exercise program around that goal.

However (here's the fine print), not everyone can be 5-foot-10 and 115 pounds. I once had a client bring in a picture of Cindy Crawford and tell me that she wanted that body. I agreed that it would be nice, but I pointed out that her bone structure didn't match—her hips were too wide, and she was too short to duplicate Cindy's body. A few things we can't change—your bones are one of them. If you measure the distance between your hip bones where they point out in front just below your waist, that's the smallest your hips can possibly be unless we go in and remove bone (which you can't do—please don't try). We can't make you taller or shorter without serious surgery; we can't make your shoulders higher or wider, your legs longer, or anything like that. What you can do is keep the bone structure you have, and sculpt the muscles on it for a knockout look.

Again, I want to remind you not to compare yourself to anyone else. We are all individuals. Sure, we all have the same muscle and bones, but we don't all look alike. That would be the same as saying that a Cadillac and a Volkswagen are the same thing because they are both cars. They both have four tires and an engine, and they both perform the same functions to get you from point A to B, but they don't look the same.

What About Metabolism?

Favorite excuse #2: "I can't get in shape because I have a slow metabolism." I just love this one. My follow-up question is always, do you know what "metabolism" is? Nobody has ever answered that question correctly, so let me define it for you. Your *metabolism* is the number of calories you burn to keep you alive. If you were to lie in bed all day and not move an inch, you would still burn calories. It takes energy to breathe, for your heart to beat and pump blood, and for your body to create enough heat to keep you warm inside. The average person burns between 1,200 and 2,000 calories every day doing nothing! If you get out of bed, get dressed, go to work or school, or move around at all, you burn more calories.

Trainer Talk

Another term for **metabolism** is your basal metabolic rate, or BMR. This is the number of calories required to keep you alive at rest, without any movement. The average person's BMR is 1,200 to 2,000 calories per day.

The misconception is that you have a slow metabolism if you don't burn everything you eat, and you end up storing some of it as fat. The problem with this "logic" is that we rarely know exactly how many calories we are eating and how many we are burning off. Do you know how many calories it takes to turn to the next page? If not, how do you know when you have eaten enough calories to accomplish that task? You don't. So we tend to eat more calories than we need to keep from running out. The problem is, any extra calories are stored as fat, and then we blame it on a slow metabolism. The fact is, your body burns calories only when it needs to. Just because you ate that 500-calorie piece of chocolate cake doesn't mean you are going to burn all those calories automatically. You have to *do* something.

Here's another way of looking at it: if we applied that same logic to your car, you would always be out of gas. Every time you put gas in your car, it would use it all up, regardless of whether you drove anywhere. Cars don't work that way, and neither does your body. Your car burns gas only when it's running or moving. Your body burns extra calories only when you move—and only as many as it needs to make it move. If you eat that piece of cake and then decide to go for a walk to "burn it off," but that walk requires only 300 calories, then you still have 200 calories to store (you really didn't burn it all off—you just don't feel so full anymore).

You also can't change your metabolism a whole lot—maybe 200 to 300 calories a day, at most. The only way to change your metabolism is to lose or gain fat weight or muscle mass. When you add fat weight, your metabolism barely moves up—just enough to help your body pump blood to the extra mass. However, when you add muscle weight, your metabolism goes up because muscle burns calories to generate heat at rest. The more muscle you gain, the more your resting metabolism increases.

If you lose fat or muscle, your metabolism goes down because your body no longer has to support that fat and there is less muscle to burn calories. The issue we run into here is that when people lose fat, they often continue to eat the same amount of food as before but with a lower metabolism rate, so more food gets stored as fat.

The point is, you shouldn't try to change your metabolism other than by increasing muscle mass. It doesn't take a lot of muscle to burn more calories at rest, but it does take work. The more you can move and exercise during the day, the more your body will burn and the less it will store (just don't start thinking you have earned that piece of cake).

Turning Fat into Muscle and Muscle into Fat

Many people believe that shaping and building muscle involves turning fat cells into muscle cells and that if you stop exercising, muscle will turn back into fat. This is a huge myth that is absolutely wrong!

Truth is, muscle and fat are two completely different tissues, and one cannot become the other. It's like saying that you can paint an apple orange and it becomes an orange. It's still an apple—with orange paint. This particular belief continues because of the perception of athletes who suddenly stop working out. When well-muscled athletes or bodybuilders decrease the intensity and amount of strenuous exercise in their lives—or stop working out altogether—they often continue to eat the same number of calories they ate during their exercising days. They are eating more than they are burning off (because they are not exercising as much anymore), so the extra calories get stored as fat.

Science Sez

Muscle and fat are not the same thing—one cannot be turned into the other. These are two completely different tissues with different chemical compositions and biological functions.

Additionally, by reducing their exercise, they inevitably lose muscle mass (decreasing their metabolic rate), giving them that flat, sagging look. Adjusting their caloric intake to match their activity level and making exercise an integral part of their lifestyle combats this scenario.

In the same light, if you carry excess body fat, you can change the composition of your body by engaging in resistance exercise. Fat is burned in the muscle, so building muscle mass helps burn off the layers of fat. It's important to remember that muscle burns calories, but fat just sits there doing nothing. If you increase the amount of active muscle you have, you burn more calories and fat. If you increase the amount of fat you have, you just get more fat. In most cases, you don't have to increase the size of your muscle to burn more fat; you just have to make the muscles you have more active. We all have muscle that is not working at its full potential for fat burning, which is why a knockout workout is so important.

Three Ways to Shape Your Body

You can change the shape of your body in lots of different ways, and there are lots of different knockout workouts to help you do that. You can make three main changes: You can make your body 1) bigger, 2) stronger, or 3) more defined. The results you get from exercise are very specific to how you train. If you want one part of your body to get stronger, but you think another just needs more definition of the muscle that is already there, you can do that. Training is specific for each muscle group and body part. You can make your arms stronger and your legs more defined, or your legs bigger and your chest more defined, or your back stronger and your arms bigger, or just about any combination you can think of. Here is how each works.

Bigger

Typically when we think of getting bigger, we think of huge, bulging muscles like those of professional bodybuilders on TV. That's definitely not what I'm talking about. Bigger muscles don't have to be preposterously huge—maybe just big enough that you can see them in the mirror. The strength of a muscle is directly related to how big it is (but that's not the only thing that makes a muscle stronger). Getting bigger muscles is a great goal if you feel that maybe your upper body is out of proportion to your lower body, or that maybe one arm is a little bigger than the other. You can focus your knockout workout to make certain parts of your body bigger with more muscle, while leaving other parts alone. Just because you train your biceps muscles to get bigger doesn't mean that your legs are going to start growing as well—that's what I mean about training being specific.

Stronger

You can gain strength without gaining size. In fact, this is what normally happens at the beginning of a new exercise program. You start off by using the muscle you already have but haven't been taking full advantage of. Every one of us has a little bit of reserve strength built into every muscle. It's this potential we want to tap into first. When you start an exercise program, you will feel the resistance get easy really quick,

even before you see any changes in the mirror. That's those muscles working their way up to full speed. When you have gotten every muscle working at its best, you can still get stronger by training it to become more efficient. Muscles are amazing structures that can learn with the help of your brain. A weight that started out taking the entire muscle to lift will eventually take only a fraction of your total muscle as you become more efficient. When you are using only part of your muscle to lift a weight that used to take all your muscle, you have some left over, so now you can lift more weight and become even stronger.

In the Mirror

The first gains in strength always occur without any apparent changes in your shape on the outside. This phenomenon is the result of your body getting smarter at using the muscle it already has to make you stronger.

More Defined

I want you to take the word *toning* out of your vocabulary because it really doesn't mean anything. Instead, replace it with *defined*. Adding definition to a muscle means that you are making its shape more apparent. Think of someone you know who has smooth, round upper arms. Now think of someone who has upper arms in which you can see the muscles—but not big muscles. That's definition. If we were to strip all the fat off your body, you would look exactly like one of the anatomy pictures you see at the beginning of Chapters 8 through 17. We all look like those pictures; we just can't see the muscle because of the layers of fat on top. When you burn off that fat and sculpt the muscles underneath, you get that defined look that tells everyone you are a knockout.

The Least You Need to Know

◆ Your body's shape is determined by what you do with it (exercise), what you feed it (nutrition), and what your parents gave you (genetics).

◆ The only way to positively affect your metabolism is to gain lean muscle.

◆ It's impossible for fat cells to turn into muscle cells, or vice versa; fat and muscle are two completely different tissues.

◆ You can increase the size of your muscles, the strength of your muscles, and how defined your muscles are.

◆ Every knockout workout will be a little different, based on your body and how you want to change it.

In This Chapter

- ◆ Change is good
- ◆ Looking great from any angle
- ◆ When, what, and how many
- ◆ Finding the right equipment
- ◆ Progressing in circles
- ◆ Change your goals—and set new ones

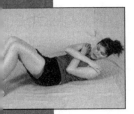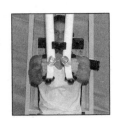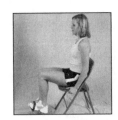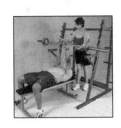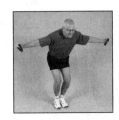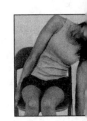

Building Your Knockout Workout

Okay, you've got the who (you) and why (because you want to), so now we've got to cover the when, what, and how many. Exercise prescription is part science and part art. The science side is always changing for the better. The more research is done, the more we know about how the body responds to exercise, and the more precise we can get with our programs. You will learn enough of the science side of things to give your program a serious edge up on the competition in the gym. This is way beyond what you will read in any magazine, but it's simple enough that you can put it to use without a degree in exercise science.

The art side of the equation is a little more tricky. In reality, a lot of trial and error is involved in finding what works the best, along with a little guesstimating when it comes time to change your program. It's not as random as picking exercises out of a hat; the art side takes a little learning and some education to make it all fit together. This chapter gives you all the info you need to know to get it right without wasting any time. After all, life is short, and you're ready to feel great and show off that new body.

Change Your Workout

Take a moment and flip through the last half of this book. See all those exercises? That's just the tip of the iceberg. Because of the sheer volume of exercises out there, I've included only the most common, the easiest to learn, and the most effective exercises. When you start your knockout workout, you'll have a set of exercises to get you started down that road of change. But just like a road trip in your car, you'll face the inevitable turns, twists, and the occasional moment of getting lost. The point is, your exercise program will not always be the same—it will change. I know people who have been doing the same thing for years (literally), and they wonder why they don't see any difference in their body anymore—it's because they have gotten used to their workout, and it is no longer a challenge to complete.

Your body will change only when you make it change. If your exercise program is within your current capability, your body doesn't have to change anything. When you make your body work harder than it usually does, things change. Muscles get stronger, bones get stronger, fat gets burned off, and shapes change—but only if you make it happen (maybe that's why it's called a *workout* instead of an *easyout*).

Remember that no miracle exercise can change your body overnight—it takes work. No one exercise will always be perfect for you. In fact, your body will respond and change faster if you change your exercise program now and then. You don't want to have an exercise "routine" because a routine is something that never changes. You want to have an evolving program that changes as you change, keeps up with your needs, and is always challenging your body to become better than it is.

Knowing when to change your exercise program is almost an art. You have to learn to listen to what your body is telling you about

each exercise. Because your muscles can't actually talk, you have to pay attention to how they work. When a current exercise becomes easy and is no longer much of a challenge, it's time to change something. That something can be a new exercise, more reps or weight on your current exercise, or less rest between sets—depending on your goals (we'll discuss this more in a minute). The thing is, something has to change to make the program a little harder, but not so hard that you can't do it. We are talking about baby steps here. Just a little change can make a big difference over time.

Forward, Backward, and Sideways

When you look at your body in the mirror, which angle do you look at? Do you just focus on what's right in front, or do you also turn around and check out your profile and what's behind you? I'm guessing you want to see everything, so you crane your neck to check out every square inch of skin you can. Well, that's good because the rest of the world sees you from many different angles as well.

Your exercise program should be built on the same principle: movement in every direction. You don't want exercises that make just the front of you look good, or just the back, or just the sides. You want the whole package.

Different exercises focus on different muscles that move in different directions. It doesn't get any more different than that! If you pay attention to how you move in a normal day, you'll see that you walk forward, step to the side, and occasionally back up. You also twist, bend, reach, stretch, and jump. We move in a lot of directions just to get around this world, so our exercises should help us navigate life with ease and good looks. You will have exercises in your program that are done sitting, standing, lying, and moving in odd directions. Everything you do increases the effectiveness of your knockout workout and enhances the results you ultimately get.

If you read some of the popular exercise magazines, especially the ones geared toward bodybuilding, you'll find that most of those exercises are designed to improve how you look facing straight on. Anyone who competes in bodybuilding is interested mostly in how they look to a judge sitting right in front of them while they are standing in one place. This isn't you, and it certainly isn't real life. We aren't trying to give you huge muscles; you want muscles that give you just the right amount of attention and strength. We're looking for muscles that are designed and trained to move and that help you look good while you move.

All the Puzzle Pieces

Putting together your knockout workout is a fairly simple process. The whole workout is made up of a few small components. Each of these components makes a different contribution to how your body will look in the end. Next I describe each item and tell you how to choose what works best for you.

The Schedule

I've often heard that you have to exercise every day for it to be effective. This is flat-out wrong. Think of it like this: anything is better than nothing, and something will get you somewhere. It's a little vague, but it makes a point. Any exercise that is more than you normally do will make a difference, even if it is just once a week. Once a week is better than zero times a week. If we keep following this logic, then twice a week is better than once, three times is better than two, four times is better than three, and so on. Fortunately, here is where science comes to our rescue. The majority of research shows that the optimal number of times for exercise in a week is three or four, which leaves you with a few days to rest and play.

Now, that being said, let me emphasize that three to four workouts a week is optimal, but not absolutely necessary. If you are just starting out and haven't been exercising already, one to two days a week is fine. Later you can add a third day, and later a fourth day. Remember what I said about baby steps! Jumping from no exercise to three to four days a week is one of the worst things you can do (and if you have ever tried that, you know what I mean). You'll be sore and tired, and you could hurt yourself. Your body has to adapt to this new stress on your muscles, so let it happen gradually.

Increasing the number of days you work out is a great way to change your program when you start reaching a plateau. If the two days a week you have been doing isn't a challenge anymore, and your body has stopped responding, add a third day. You've just increased your total weekly exercise by 50 percent—that ought to get the ball rolling again.

Now, some people work out every day of the week, and that's okay. This type of training takes some time to get used to and has to be done very carefully so that your muscles get enough rest between workouts (more on this in a moment). I don't normally recommend daily training unless you are getting ready for some type of athletic competition or you are dividing one workout into smaller parts because of a tight schedule. With this approach, it's best to split the weight training and cardio work between different days, alternating weight training one day and cardio the next. But even then, a day of rest every three to four days will actually give you more results than working out every day. It's actually during rest that your body is able to recover and get stronger.

So Many Exercises, So Little Time

Now that you have exercise scheduled into your daily activities, we need to focus on what exactly you will be doing during those days. This book has approximately 150 exercises, with all the variations, so it makes sense that you can't do everything. That would be one long workout! So we have to narrow the field a little.

You can approach your workout in a couple of ways: 1) the full-body workout or 2) the split workout. A full-body workout includes at least one exercise for every body part. A split workout works only part of your body, saving the other part for another workout. The benefit of a full-body workout is that you get everything done in one session. The benefit of the split workout is that it allows you to do two to three exercises for each muscle group because you work half of your muscles in one workout. This gives you more time to focus on each part of your body.

Here's an example of a full-body workout that you can do every other day:

- ◆ Crunch
- ◆ Wall Press
- ◆ Pull-Up
- ◆ Front Raise
- ◆ Machine Curl
- ◆ Kickback
- ◆ Superman Squeeze
- ◆ Wall Squat
- ◆ Lying Machine Curl
- ◆ Calf-Raise Machine

Here's an example of a split workout that's divided between two consecutive days:

Day 1:

- ◆ Oblique
- ◆ Push-Up
- ◆ Chin-Up
- ◆ Lateral Raise
- ◆ Preacher Curl

Day 2:

- ◆ Overhead Press
- ◆ Lying Leg Lift
- ◆ Dumbbell Squat
- ◆ Seated Machine Curls
- ◆ Seated Calf Raise

The major factor that determines how many exercises you should include in a workout is how much time you have. It's easy to pick out 15 exercises, but if you have only 20 minutes for your workout, you won't be able to finish. It may take a little trial and error to determine how many exercises you can fit into your schedule. Of course, more is better, but don't ignore one body part so you can work another muscle a little more. You need to keep a balanced approach, lest you become lopsided. In the next chapter, I provide some starter workouts that are designed to take up 30 minutes a day.

On the Level

I've also categorized all the exercises based on the level of intensity they provide:

- ◆ *Level 1 exercises* are great for beginners and staple exercises that will always get your heart rate up.
- ◆ *Level 2 exercises* are a little more advanced, increase the intensity a little more, require some basic strength in that area, and a mastery of the level 1 exercises.
- ◆ *Levels 3* and *4 exercises* are advanced exercises that will push your body as far as possible. Only attempt level 3 or 4 exercises after you have mastered any level 1 or 2 exercises in the same muscle group.

Repeated Fun

When you have chosen the exercises you want to do, the next question is how many repetitions (reps) of each exercise are appropriate. It depends on your goal. If you want to improve your strength, complete one to six repetitions per set (more on sets in a minute). If your goal is to make a muscle bigger, finish 7 to 12 reps. If you are focusing on *definition* and building *muscular endurance*, 13 to 18 reps is for you.

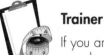

Trainer Talk _____

If you are training for **definition**, you are also building **muscular endurance**; therefore, these terms can be used interchangeably.

The more repetitions you do for each exercise, the longer your workout will take and the fewer exercises you can do in one workout. For instance, it takes half the amount of time to complete 8 repetitions of 8 exercises (training to get bigger) than it does to complete 16 repetitions of 8 exercises (training for definition). So the number of exercises is a factor in not only how long your workout lasts, but also how many reps you do of each exercise.

Setting Yourself Up

The next component is the number of sets you complete of each exercise. A set can have anywhere from 1 to 18 repetitions in it, depending on your goal. The best place to start if you are a beginner is to complete one set of each exercise in your program. When that gets easy, or when you have more time, add a second set. Go to three sets when two is no longer a problem and you want more results. Increasing the number of sets beyond three per exercise hasn't really been shown to be very useful because of the law of diminishing returns. When you move up

from one set to two, you double the amount of exercise you are doing (100 percent increase). But when you move from two sets to three, the exercise is increased by only 50 percent. A fourth set would be only a 33 percent increase, a fifth set would be a 25 percent increase, and it goes down from there. Additionally, the benefit you get each time you increase the number of sets is only about half of the amount of work you do. So if you double the amount of work by moving from one set to two, you are only going to get about 50 percent more benefit. After the third set, the benefits are less than 15 percent, which isn't much for all that extra work.

Spot Me _____

Never—I repeat, *never*—start a new exercise with more than one set. Your body needs time to get adjusted to the new stimulus, and more than one set will probably make you sore (which doesn't mean anything good has happened).

Not Too Little, Not Too Much

Ready to work out now? Let's see: you know what days you will exercise, you've picked out what exercises to do, you know how many sets and reps to do … so what's left? Oh, right—the weight. That's pretty important! Choosing the correct weight or resistance for each exercise has a huge impact on the results you get. Fortunately, this part is easy. The amount of weight you use is based on your goal—and, more specifically, the number of reps you are supposed to do. To recap, here are the number of reps for each goal:

- ◆ Strength = 1–6 reps
- ◆ Size = 7–12 reps
- ◆ Definition = 13–18 reps

The amount of weight you can lift and the number of times you can lift it are inversely proportional (I just like using big words now and then). This basically means that the more weight you use, the fewer number of times you can lift it. The less weight you use, the greater number of times you can lift it. Here's an example: pick up a pencil and raise it over your head. Now lower it back to your side. Repeat this as many times as you can, or until you get bored (I bet you get bored first). Now find something heavier, such as a big rock or a gallon of milk. See how many times you can lift it over your head. I'll bet you didn't lift the rock as many times as you did the pencil. Why? Because the rock weighs more. The heavier something is, the fewer times you can lift it. If it's light enough, you can lift it all day. And of course, nobody ever saw a change in their body from just lifting a pencil.

To find the right weight for your goals, find a weight that you can lift for at least the minimum number of reps, but no more than the maximum number of reps. If you can lift it more than the maximum number of reps, increase the weight. If you can't get the minimum number of reps, decrease the weight. Some trial and error is involved (again, the art of exercise prescription), but it's easy.

The Right Equipment

What's the difference between lifting a 10-pound dumbbell and a 10-pound turkey? Give up? There is no difference—they both weigh 10 pounds. Commercial gyms and health clubs would have you believe that you have to use big, fancy equipment to get a good workout. That's a bunch of baloney. If it has weight, you can use it for exercise. It doesn't have to be big and shiny, or have the latest contraption attached to it. In fact, the best piece of resistance equipment in the world is free—it's called gravity. Gravity gives everything weight. So that gallon

milk jug is a perfect dumbbell (you can even adjust the weight by drinking the milk).

Throughout Part 3, you will see a variety of equipment used. I developed many of the exercises simply by choosing the most effective moves that require the least amount of equipment. Most of the time, dumbbells, resistance tubing, your own body weight, and maybe a stability ball is all you need. A few exercises require special equipment, but not very many. When special gym equipment is the best choice, I've tried to provide a variation so you don't have to join a gym to do the exercise.

Spot Me

If you will be exercising at home, it's important to get good-quality equipment. Don't go for the cheapest equipment on the market because you do get what you pay for. Cheap, low-grade equipment may save you a few bucks in the beginning, but you will have to replace it often. And there is nothing good about a resistance band snapping or a stability ball popping. Shop for and buy your equipment from a reputable sporting goods store or online merchant instead of a department store that doesn't know much about the equipment. See Appendix B for some good resources.

Moving Forward

Progression is one of the key elements of a successful knockout workout program. Without progression, you will maintain what you have but never improve. And what's the point of working out if you are not going to make improvements? I know you don't want to become one of those people who gets stuck in the same routine for years, never making any progress. Here's a way to ensure that every workout moves you closer to your goal.

The key to progression lies in always giving 100 percent effort on every repetition of every set of every exercise in every workout. Progression is all about taking baby steps, never any big leaps. The idea is that you always push your exercise program just a little bit further than before. That makes your body push itself a little further, and it gets you ever closer to your goals.

Trainer Talk

Progression refers to consistently intensifying your workout so that it remains a challenge and brings continual improvements.

The first step of progression lies in the smallest component of your program: the repetitions. Remember those ranges of repetitions for each goal? I didn't specify a particular number of reps; I gave you a range of reps. Ranges are important because they are open-ended. If I gave you the exercise prescription of 10 reps, you would do 10 reps and stop. But what if you were able to do 11 or 12? Well, you stopped at 10, so your body wasn't able to work to its potential, which means you probably won't see much improvement. That's not what we want! You want to move forward, not stay where you're at. Ranges of repetitions allow you to push yourself.

Remember what I said about the weight you should use? The weight depends on the repetitions. Choose a weight that allows you to do at least the minimum number of reps for your goal, but no more than the maximum number of reps. When you put these two components together, you have a way of moving your workouts forward: circular progression.

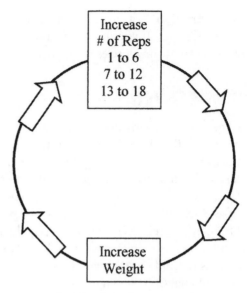

Principle of circular progression.

For example, if you are working on definition (a rep range of 13 to 18), your goal every set should be to get 18 reps, the maximum for this goal. When you can do this maximum number for two consecutive workouts, increase the weight the next time. When you add more weight, you probably won't be able to get 18 reps again, but that's fine; as long as you can get at least 13, you are still on track. Keep working with that weight until you can do it 18 reps for two workouts; then move it up again. This pattern of progressing through the range of repetitions and then adding weight keeps you moving forward because you are always pushing yourself toward the next goal. When you reach that goal, you move the goal a little further and start toward it again. The same example works for building strength or getting bigger: always push toward the maximum number of reps for your goal, and when you reach it, add more weight and begin again. That's why it's called circular progression.

Over time, as you get closer to your goals, it will take longer to reach the top of the repetition range, and you won't increase the weight very often. That's fine, as long as you are always pushing yourself to do as many repetitions as you can in each set. If you do this, you will always stimulate your muscles to improve.

You've Arrived

I love the question "How long will it take me to get in shape?" Boy, I wish I knew the answer to that one. I've been working out for more than 15 years and still haven't reached my full potential. I have reached several goals and then set new ones. Over the course of my years as a personal trainer, I've seen many clients reach their goals and then move on to new ones. I've also seen clients reach their goals and then start in with a maintenance program just to stay where they were.

How do you know when you've arrived at your destination? If you start with a particular look or goal in mind, that makes it easy. However, if your goal is just to improve, you will probably meet your goal within just a few workouts—but I doubt you'll be ready to stop. You see, every workout causes an improvement, even if it isn't one you can see in a mirror. Your goals may change as you change. Some of my clients started out to lose weight and then noticed that they were getting stronger. So they worked on that for a while and decided that they wanted more definition from their newfound muscles, so their goal changed again. Absolutely nothing is wrong with changing your goals and making new ones. In fact, I'll bet that's one of the best ways to keep yourself motivated. Just keep pushing that goal further away so you keep working. Fitness is an elusive thing that can't be held without work. Once you reach a goal, you can't stop or you'll move backward—you might as well move forward!

If you need a tool to help you in your quest, use a journal. I recommend that all my clients and students journal workouts. If you wonder how far you've come, just flip back a few pages and see your progress. You can chart every set of every workout you do in a spiral notebook so you can easily find a past workout. This is a great way to track progress and see the numbers change on paper while you change in the mirror.

The Least You Need to Know

◆ Your body changes only when you make it change—an exercise has to be more than you are used to, or there is no reason for your body to adapt.

◆ An exercise program should work every muscle possible because there is more to you than what you can see in the mirror.

◆ Training for increased muscle size, definition, or strength involves different amounts of repetitions and weight.

◆ Progression is an ongoing process that allows you to keep making changes in your workout at the appropriate times.

◆ Your goals can be dynamic and changing. No rule says that you cannot change your mind midworkout—change is actually a good thing.

In This Chapter

- ◆ Developing a game plan
- ◆ Basic workouts that target problem areas, add definition, and build strength
- ◆ Exercise plans for pre- and post-pregnancy
- ◆ Workouts to strengthen your core muscles
- ◆ Keeping your motivation high
- ◆ The benefits of working with a personal trainer

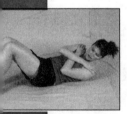 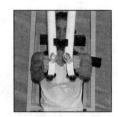 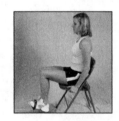 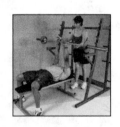 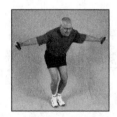 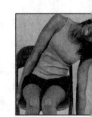

Chapter 4

Knock Their Socks Off

Pick up any fitness magazine, and you're likely to see one of these headlines: "Secret workouts of the stars revealed," "Top ten exercises to tone those flabby arms," "Banish that belly with these awesome moves," or "No time, no problem—world's fastest workout for you." Every single month, year after year, I keep seeing the same exercise plans. I don't have a problem with magazines printing exercises—hopefully someone will buy them and actually do the exercises. What I do have a problem with is one-size-fits-all exercise plans that don't deliver. Like I always say, there are no secret workouts, no "special" exercises, and definitely no shortcuts to getting a knockout body.

What I can promise you is that there is always more than one way to reach your goals. One route gets you there slowly because it isn't focused on what you need. Another route is really effective because it works on only what you need to work on. Simple is always better, and a plan may have more than the "top ten" exercises in one plan. This chapter gives you the direction to get you started on the road to a knockout workout. Get ready to discover what you need to do to get the results you seek.

What's Your Game Plan?

By now you understand the basics of how to put together a knockout workout that will work for you. You have a good idea of what you want your body to look like—picture that in your mind. You also know about how much time you have to work out every day, how many sets and reps you need to complete, and how to keep your program moving forward using circular progression, which I discussed in Chapter 3. In case you've suffered a bit of information overload so far, here's a recap:

◆ **Number of workouts each week:** 1–4, depending on how advanced you are, and as long as you aren't sore

◆ **Number of exercises:** As many as you can safely fit into the time you have (the more, the better)

◆ **Number of sets:** 1–3, starting with 1 and building up to 3

◆ **Number of reps:** Depends on your goal: More strength = 1–6, increased muscle size = 7–12, more defined muscles = 13–16

However, I'm not going to just leave you with that—there is still too much to do. Given what you know now, you could put together any number of different workouts, but do you know the best route to your goals? It's time you developed a *game plan*—kind of like a system to make sure you are using the right exercises for your body. If you ask a dozen football coaches about their game plan, you'll probably get a dozen different answers, even though they all have the same goal: to win the game. Each coach's game plan is based on what he has to work with and what his players are capable of. A good game plan for a basketball team may be to slam-dunk the ball every time they get it—that way, there won't be any missed shots. Sounds good, right? But what if nobody on the team is tall enough to dunk? That game plan, as good as it sounds, just won't work.

Trainer Talk

A **game plan** is a personalized guide for your knockout workout. It details the exercises you are going to do, how much of them you will do, and when you will do them. Keep a good record of your game plan in your workout journal so you can refer to it from time to time to judge your progress.

Remember in Chapter 3 when I said that an exercise prescription is part science and part art? This is the part of the plan in which a lot of art is needed. There's no way for me to list a workout for every possible person out there. Exercise is too individual for that (which is why the magazine workouts don't usually work). You have to use the information you have learned so far, and what you know about your body, to start designing your workout. And this will change. No workout is perfect the first time (even the ones I write). You have to watch how your body responds to each exercise and make adjustments based on that. If something works, stick with it. If it isn't giving you what you want, change it. It's that simple. But (there is always a but) don't change things too fast. You have to give an exercise time to make a difference. One week, or even one month, usually isn't long enough to tell if something doesn't work (unless the exercise is painful—then one day is enough). Don't base your exercise choices on how much it makes you sore. Soreness isn't a good thing and is not a way to determine whether an exercise works.

Put together a plan that includes exercises that target the areas you want to work (a few of my favorite workouts are coming up), try it for about six to eight weeks, and then make adjustments. Try not to scrap the entire workout, but change just a few exercises at a time. It should be a modification, not a new start. Then work with that for six to eight weeks and modify it again. Keep making modifications as needed. After a while, the exercises that worked in the beginning may get boring or may lose their effectiveness as your body changes. Add more challenging exercises to keep your body guessing what's next.

Your game plan should be yours alone. It's fine to work out with a partner, but that person's program will be different even if you have the same goal because your bodies are different. Get feedback from your friends. Ask them how they think your body is changing. You know how the fans always see things that the coaches and referees miss? Same thing here. Look at yourself in the mirror, feel how your body is changing, and ask your friends what they think—and tell them to be honest. Your game plan will always lead you to victory if you are adaptable and keep pushing forward—consider this a slam-dunk!

In the Mirror

Ask your friends and family for their honest opinions of how your workout is working. You have to find people who won't feed you the "you look fine just the way you are" line. If you were content with the way you looked, you wouldn't be reading this book. It may sometimes hurt, but candid feedback can be your best weapon in creating a knockout workout.

Basic Workout Plans

Chances are, someone else out there has the same goals and the same knockout look in their mind. In the 18 years I've been training people—and I'm talking about hundreds of people—I sometimes think I've seen it all (but every now and then I'm surprised). A few goals seem to be the most popular—with losing weight being at the top of the list—so I've put together what I think are some pretty darn good workouts to help you get started if your goals are similar to one of these.

I've always liked the phrase "don't reinvent the wheel," and I use it often in my own training.

When I have a client with a goal that I haven't heard before, I don't try to design a workout from scratch. I call some of my colleagues to ask their advice (this is a sign of a good trainer, by the way—one who doesn't pretend to know everything about everyone). I gather as much information as I can about the goal, including what has worked for some people and what hasn't worked, and I use that to help me design an individual workout for my client.

The following workouts are some basic starting points for you to build on. These are the long versions for those of you who are a bit more advanced. If you are a beginner, start with just one or two days a week, and just one or two sets of each exercise until you build your way up to more. You don't even have to use the whole workout to get results. When you reach the advanced stages, feel free to make modifications to fit you. These are great starting points designed to give you an idea of the kind of exercises that will focus your game plan a little.

Banish That Belly

When I think back to every person I've trained describing their goal to me, most of them grabbed their stomach fat and said they wanted to "get rid of this." The first thing you need to understand about losing stomach fat is that you can't isolate just that part of your body. When you lose fat, it comes off your entire body, not just any one area. However, because you have more fat in certain areas, you will notice that those areas change the most. This is my favorite plan for banishing that extra belly fat:

- **Monday:** 30 minutes of cardio
- **Tuesday:** Two sets of 13–16 reps of Crunches, Tubing Presses, Tubing Rows, Dumbbell Squats, Upright Rows, and Step-Ups
- **Thursday:** 40 minutes of cardio

◆ **Friday:** Three sets of 13–16 reps of Obliques, Kickbacks, Leaning Bridge, Toe Press, Tubing Curl, and Front Raise

◆ **Saturday:** 30 minutes of cardio

Leave That Fat Behind

The second most common area where people want to lose weight is their backside (also known as your behind, buttocks, butt, etc.). Just like stomach fat, we can't just lose backside fat, but we can work out in ways that will make the fat burn and define the muscles more. Here's my plan for a supreme sitting area:

◆ **Monday:** 30 minutes of cardio

◆ **Tuesday:** Two sets of 13–16 reps of Lying Leg Lift, Donkey Kicks, Dumbbell Squat, Machine Press, and Lat Pulldown

◆ **Thursday:** 40 minutes of cardio

◆ **Friday:** Three sets of 13–16 reps of Crunches, Seated Press, Dumbbell Curl, Leg Press, Lying Machine Curl, Standing and Lateral Lift

◆ **Saturday:** 30 minutes of cardio

Saddlebags Are for Horses

A certain celebrity has actually made most of her fortune selling an exercise device that's supposed to slim down and shape up your hips. But just because she had nice hips doesn't mean that machine did it. It takes more than just one exercise to target the fat in this area, so here's my hippest workout ever:

◆ **Monday:** 30 minutes of cardio

◆ **Tuesday:** Two sets of 13–16 reps of Superman Squeeze, Walking Lunge, Overhead Press, Hammer Curl, Lean Forward, Stair Press

◆ **Thursday:** 40 minutes of cardio

◆ **Friday:** Three sets of 13–16 reps of Standing Pushback, Stomp, Dumbbell Press, Tubing Press, Tubing Row

◆ **Saturday:** 30 minutes of cardio

Definition Beyond the Dictionary

So you've got some muscle, but you aren't happy with how it looks. You want people to look at you and instantly think, "Wow, check out those muscles—that's cool!" I know how you feel. After all this hard work, you want it to show without you having to flex all the time. Your muscles want to be defined, too—that's their nature. Here is a great full-body shaping routine to give you that sculpted look:

◆ **Monday:** 15 minutes of cardio; two sets of 13–16 reps of Calf-Raise Machine, Leg Press, Preacher Curl, Lat Pulldown, Leg-Extension Machine, Seated Machine Curl, Concentration Curl, and Tubing Row

◆ **Tuesday:** 30 minutes of cardio, one set of 7–12 reps of Dumbbell Press, Lateral Raise, Standing Pushdown, Machine Press, Upright Row, and French Curl

◆ **Thursday:** 15 minutes of cardio; two sets of 13–16 reps of Triceps-Press Machine, Shoulder-Press Machine, and Push-Ups

◆ **Friday:** 30 minutes of cardio; one set of 7–12 reps of Leg Press, Standing Curl, Bent-Over Row, EZ Bar Curl, Seated Calf Raise, Wall Squat, Reverse Curl, Lying Pull-Up

Lifting for Upper-Body Strength

Did you know that, pound for pound, men's and women's lower body strength is equal, but women's upper-body strength is lower (generally, that is)? This is an area I see a lot of women interested in, but I'm not forgetting about the guys. Regardless of gender, increasing upper-body strength follows the same rules for sets and reps. Here are some favorite getting-stronger exercises, using a split program with two workouts each day:

- **Monday morning:** Two sets of 1–6 reps of Crunches, Bench Press, Pullover, Front Raise, and Angled Raise
- **Monday evening:** One set of 1–6 reps of Crunches, Bench Press, Pullover, Front Raise, and Angled Raise
- **Wednesday morning:** Two sets of 1–6 reps of Sit-Ups, Preacher Curl, Lying Press, Inline Press, and Bent-Over Row
- **Wednesday evening:** Two sets of 1–6 reps of Burner Abs, Push-Ups, Lat Pulldown, and Military Press
- **Friday morning:** Two sets of 1–6 reps of Overhead Press, Hammer Curl, Kickbacks, Low-Pulley Curl, Sit-Ups, and Tubing Press
- **Friday evening:** One set of 1–6 reps of Crunches, Straight-Arm Pulldown, Dumbbell Fly, and Barbell Raise

Pushing for Lower-Body Strength

Your legs mainly push you through life. Their main job is stepping, jumping, climbing, and seeing that you get off the couch to go work out. Stronger legs are always a great asset, especially if you have a job or lifestyle that requires you to be on your feet all day. Follow this split workout if you want the strongest legs on the block:

- **Monday morning:** Two sets of 1–6 reps of Stomp, Dumbbell Squat, Lean Forward, Calf-Raise Machine, and Step-Ups
- **Monday evening:** One set of 1–6 reps of Barbell Squat, Standing Pushback, Leg-Extension Machine, and Lying Machine Curl

- **Wednesday morning:** Two sets of 1–6 reps of Stair Press, Wall Squat, Walking Lunge, and Seated Machine Curl
- **Wednesday evening:** Two sets of 1–6 reps of Lying Leg Lift, Donkey Kick, and Barbell Squat
- **Friday morning:** Two sets of 1–6 reps of Walking Lunge, Standing Curl, Glute-Press Machine, Stomp, and Wall Squat
- **Friday evening:** One set of 1–6 reps of Toe Press, Lying Bridge, Dumbbell Squat, Stair Press, Seated Machine Curl, Standing Pushback, and Leg Press

Gearing Up for Pregnancy

Deciding to have a baby is not only a big emotional decision, but it's also a huge strain on your body. Before you make the leap toward motherhood, let's get your body ready for the trials and tolls that growing a baby entails. This workout should not be started after you are already pregnant—this is a getting-ready-to-get-pregnant workout to prepare your body. I call this my baby-body prep routine:

- **Monday/Wednesday/Friday:** 30 minutes of cardio; one set of 13–16 reps of Crunches, Reverse Crunches, Incline Press, Lying Pull-Up, Seated Press, EZ Bar Curl, Standing Pushdown, Lying Leg Lift, Dumbbell Squat, Lying Bridge, and Toe Press
- **Tuesday/Thursday:** Two sets of 7–12 reps of Leg Press, Lying Machine Curl, Sit-Ups, Push-Ups, Lat Pulldown, and Burner Abs

Spot Me

If you are already pregnant, be sure to consult your doctor before beginning any new exercise routine—the extra stress of a new workout could be too much.

Reclaiming Your Body After Pregnancy

I had a lady tell me she wanted to lose the weight she gained during pregnancy and get back to her previous shape. I asked her how old her child was, and she said 13! That's a little more postpartum than I was thinking, but hey, it's never too late to get into shape. This workout is for you gals who just had that baby and are ready to get back into your favorite jeans:

- **Monday:** 15 minutes of cardio; two sets of 13–16 reps of Crunches, Reverse Crunches, Push-Ups, and Lying Pull-Ups
- **Tuesday:** 15 minutes of cardio; two sets of 13–16 reps of Wall Squat, Concentration Curl, Kickback, and Seated Press
- **Thursday:** 20 minutes of cardio; two sets of 7–12 reps of Sit-Ups, Dumbbell Squat, Donkey Kick, and Tubing Press
- **Friday:** 30 minutes of cardio; one set of 7–12 reps of Seated Row, Obliques, Stomp, and Seated Calf Raise
- **Saturday:** 30 minutes of cardio; two sets of 13–16 reps of Double Tuck

Stable Core for a Strong Back

Got back pain? About 7 out of 10 people do sometime in their life. Been there, done that. It wasn't fun, so I designed what I think is a most excellent workout for strengthening all those muscles in your core, from your hips to your neck. A stable core is the key to holding all those vertebrae in just the right place:

- **Monday/Wednesday:** Two sets of 7–12 reps of Double Tuck, Seated Row, Reverse Crunches, Lying Pull-Ups, and Dumbbell Fly
- **Tuesday/Thursday:** Two sets of 7–12 reps of Superman Squeeze, Bent-Over Row, Crunches, Straight-Arm Pulldown, and Tubing Row
- **Saturday:** One set of 13–16 reps of Lat Pulldown, Sit-Ups, Pullover, and Push-Ups

Spot Me

Make sure you aren't experiencing any back pain before you begin this exercise, and consult your doctor if you are unsure. If you have had back pain in the past (but not now), start slowly and increase your reps when you are comfortable your body can handle it.

Incredible Abdominals

Yes, this will take more than 3 minutes a day—sorry. Probably the most advertised body part in the world is your abdominals, which I find funny because it's usually covered by your shirt (unless you live at the beach or work in late-night infomercials). But maybe you do go to the beach a lot or just want to be able to show off your abs at parties. Whatever your reason, here is a workout designed to make that stomach burn:

- **Monday:** One set of 13–16 reps of Crunches, Reverse Crunches, Sit-Ups, Crunches (again), Reverse Crunches (again), Sit-Ups (again), and Burner Abs
- **Tuesday:** Two sets of 13–16 reps of Double Tuck, Inclined Roll, and Obliques
- **Wednesday:** One set of 13–16 reps of Obliques, Sit-Ups, Obliques (again), Double Tuck, Obliques (again), and Burner Abs
- **Friday:** Three sets of 13–16 reps of Inclined Roll, Crunches, Reverse Crunches, Crunches (again), and Burner Abs

Staying Motivated

Maintaining the excitement and motivation that you have at the beginning of your program can be a challenge. Inevitably there will be times when you aren't motivated to keep up with your workouts—and that's okay. You need to recognize that sometimes life's challenges will get in the way and something has to give. The key to temporary setbacks is this: remember that you can always jump back into your program. As your knockout workout becomes part of your daily life, you won't be so quick to toss it aside when time gets short. It will become as natural as any of your other daily obligations, such as taking time to walk the dog or clean the house. Though it may seem difficult to imagine right now, there will come a time when you have difficulty skipping a workout. Exercise will become a part of your life that is always positive, always beneficial, and always just for you.

If your motivation wanes, think back to why you started in the first place, and look back to your workout journal—then you'll see the progress you have made and that will give you the boost you need. Because your goals may change as you go along, your motivation will increase as you meet one goal and set the next. Above all else, remember that you can reach each of your goals with patience and hard work. The body is an instrument that can be molded into whatever you want it to be, as long as you keep working with it.

In the Mirror

Even if you miss a few days or even a few weeks of your workout because of life's inevitable challenges, don't give up—you can go back to your body-sculpting routine at any time. You may not be able to pick up exactly where you left off, so drop back just a little on the reps or weight to get your body used to the movement again.

Working with a Pro

From time to time, I suggest that you meet with a professional personal trainer to give your program a boost. Even I, as a personal trainer, use other trainers and coaches to give me a kick in the pants from time to time, to push myself

to new levels. A personal trainer can help you measure your progress, assist you in evaluating whether you are doing exercises correctly, and provide you with another means of motivation. I always want to give my trainer or coach a positive report when I see them—it pushes me to reach new goals and keep working harder.

You don't have to work with a trainer all the time. Once every few weeks, or even once a month for a program checkup, is fine. You can find a professional personal trainer by calling your local fitness center, looking in the phone book under "Personal Training," or asking friends for referrals. Look for a trainer who is certified by the National Strength and Conditioning Association (the top certification for personal trainers) or the American College of Sports Medicine (most often found working in hospital-based fitness centers). See Appendix B for information on both of these organizations.

The Least You Need to Know

◆ You can reach your goal in many different ways, so changing your exercise program is fine—even preferred.

◆ It's important to develop a game plan to customize your workout to your needs and your body. You don't have to make up your program from scratch; you can improve upon the work that someone else did.

◆ Whether you want to lose weight in general, tone up a specific area, build strength, or accomplish something else, there's a workout that targets that goal.

◆ It's okay to take a day or two off from your workouts now and then—you won't lose that much ground, and you may even recuperate from your workouts better.

◆ Occasionally employ the services of a professional personal trainer to evaluate your program and give you a little motivational kick in the pants.

In This Part

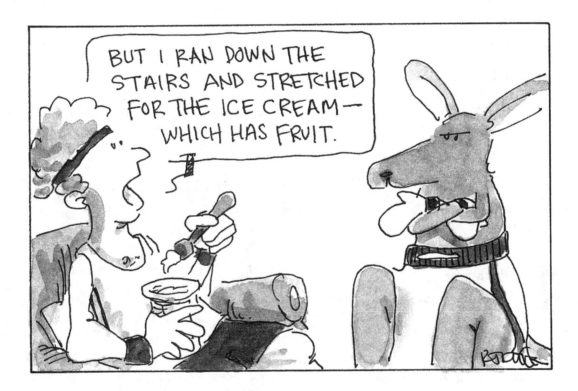

2

The Well-Rounded Approach

Getting that knockout look will take a little more than just resistance training. To make sure you cover every aspect of personal fitness, you have to include more than just working your muscles. The middle part of this book fills in all the extra pieces of your plan so that nothing is left out. Here you will learn about cardiovascular exercise for that most important muscle in your body, the heart; how to increase and maintain flexibility so every move you make is fluid and feels good; and the basic ingredients of proper nutrition to give your body the fuel to build that knockout look.

In This Chapter

◆ The most important muscle in your body

◆ What it takes to lose a pound a week

◆ Mix it up with aerobic exercise and resistance training

◆ Two ways to determine the intensity of an aerobic workout

◆ Indoor and outdoor aerobic options

◆ The importance of cooling down

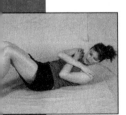
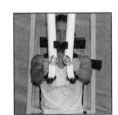
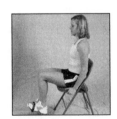
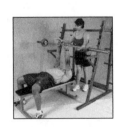
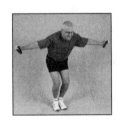
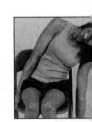

Chapter 5

The Cardio Component

 If the first thing that comes to your mind when I say "cardiovascular exercise" is a picture of yourself sweating it out on a treadmill for hours on end, you've got the wrong idea. It has nothing to do with sweat. Smelly gym clothes aside, cardiovascular exercise (also called aerobic exercise) is all about working the most important muscle you have: your heart. In fact, your heart is your body's primary muscle—without it, nothing else works! Think about that. Now you understand why it's so important to keep it strong.

   We usually don't even think about our heart beating—it's pretty automatic. Imagine if you had to consciously think about making your heart beat, like you have to think about turning the page. You couldn't ever sleep! The heart is an amazing structure that is essentially a big muscle that squeezes blood through the body when it contracts. Aerobic exercise will not only help you build a strong heart, but it will also help you burn calories—which will help you lose fat and increase your endurance, which will help you make it through all those fun and exciting knockout workouts! See, it's way more than sweating.

Time to Burn Some Fat

The most common question I get concerning aerobic exercise is "How much?" Most professional health and fitness organizations recommend between 20 and 60 minutes of aerobic exercise on most days of the week. How much time you spend on the aerobic part of your program is really a function of how much time you have, how intense you want to work, and what your goals are.

In the Mirror

Resistance training alone won't give you the ultimate knockout look. Aerobic exercise is the best way to burn fat, while resistance training is the best way to define your muscles. It doesn't do any good to have defined muscles if you can't see them because a layer of fat is hiding that shape. Combine aerobic and resistance training for the best results.

One of the most common excuses I hear from people who don't do any aerobic exercise is "I don't have enough time." But it's easier than you might think. If you are lucky enough to have a solid hour that you can devote to aerobic exercise, kudos to you. If you don't have an hour to work out all at once, divide your exercise into smaller parts. Doing two 30-minute sessions or four 15-minute sessions is just as beneficial as working out for a solid hour. It doesn't matter how many calories you burn all at once, as long as you burn them. A few minutes here and a few there adds up to a lot of calories burned—just like eating a little here and a little there adds up to a lot of calories stored.

The harder or more intense you work at your aerobic exercise, the less time it takes to burn the calories you need. This part is common sense: if you work harder and move your muscles faster, you burn more calories. For example, you'll burn more calories jogging for a half-hour than walking for a half-hour. And every little bit helps—if you drove when you could have ridden your bike, or took the elevator instead of the stairs, it will take longer to reach your goals.

The final factor in deciding how much time you spend on the aerobic part of your program is your individual goal. If you need to burn off some extra fat, here's the rule: to lose a pound of fat, you have to burn off 3,500 calories. A good and safe rate of weight loss is 1 pound a week. So if you want to lose a pound of fat each week, you will need to burn 500 extra calories a day (3,500 divided by 7 days). I don't recommend losing more than a pound of fat each week. Not only does it take a whole lot more aerobic exercise (more time, more stress on your body, less fun), but your body can adapt to slower weight loss more easily than it can to rapid weight loss. Probably the most unknockout look you can get is the saggy skin that results from losing too much weight too fast.

When you have that knockout look, or when you're comfortable maintaining your weight without losing more fat, you can adjust your exercise routines to burn only as many calories as you eat (see Chapter 7 for more on this). This includes the calories burned from both resistance training and aerobic exercise. In reality, when you are at your target body-fat percentage, it takes very little aerobic exercise to maintain it (provided that you keep your calorie intake under control). Although the amount you need to burn may vary from day to day, try to do at least 30 minutes of aerobic activity to keep your heart in good shape.

A Daily Dose

Almost all fitness professionals recommend daily aerobic exercise, but in real life you may not have time for both aerobic and resistance training every day. So what do you do?

Fortunately, resistance training also burns calories, though not as many as an aerobic workout. If you can fit in three to four aerobic workouts each week, plus your resistance training, you will make great progress toward that knockout look. In fact, it's often a good idea to alternate your aerobic and resistance-training workouts on different days so your muscles have time to rest and recuperate between workouts. At the very minimum, two days of cardio a week will improve the strength of your heart, even if you're not burning off a lot of extra fat.

Spot Me

By alternating your daily workouts between aerobic exercise and resistance training, you'll burn calories every day, plus give your muscles time to recuperate. But be careful: doing too much exercise without enough rest can lead to injury and burnout.

Very few people (usually only advanced athletes) can handle both aerobic workouts and resistance training on a daily basis. If you're a beginner, start with a minimum of two days of cardio a week—then add another day, then another. You can gradually add more aerobic exercise by increasing the amount of time for each session, increasing the intensity of your workout, and changing the type of exercise.

Faster vs. Harder

The intensity of your aerobic exercise makes a difference in how many calories you burn during each session and how quickly you reach your goals. Though it's true that you burn calories any time you move, certain levels of exercise maximize your results without overly stressing or wearing down your body. You can determine the proper intensity in two ways:

- Use a certain percentage of your maximum heart rate
- Use a subjective measure called perceived exertion

Both methods can help you put your aerobic exercise plan into action and ensure that you are doing just the right amount of activity—not too much, not too little.

Calculate Your Heart Rate Training Zone

Because aerobic exercise is essentially a workout for your heart, it makes sense to base your intensity level on how hard your heart is working. Everybody's heart responds to exercise the same way: the harder the exercise is (pushing more weight, moving faster, using more muscles), the higher your heart rate will be. Designing your exercise program based upon heart rate is a tried-and-true method that fitness professionals have used for decades. This method is individualized based upon your age and your resting heart rate. Use the following method to calculate a heart rate range that is right for you. Here's how it works:

1. Determine your 1-minute resting heart rate. It's best to sit down and rest for a few minutes, to allow your heart rate to reach its lowest level. Measure your heart rate by using your index finger and middle finger to find your pulse on either your wrist or your neck (see the following photos for clarification). Count your pulse for 1 minute.

2. Subtract your age from 220. This is an estimate of your maximum heart rate—the highest your heart rate can possibly go with intense exercise.

3. Subtract your 1-minute resting heart rate from your maximum heart rate. The result is your heart rate reserve—the number of beats your heart rate can increase from resting to maximum effort.

4. Multiply this number by 0.6 and by 0.8 to determine 60 percent and 80 percent of your heart rate reserve.

5. You now have two numbers. Add your 1-minute resting heart rate to each of them. These numbers represent the low and high target heart rates for aerobic exercise intensity—a.k.a. your heart rate training zone.

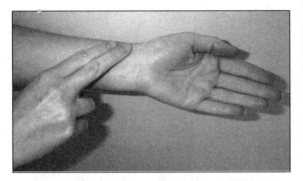

Use your index finger and middle finger to find your pulse at your wrist. Your pulse point is in the groove just below your palm on the thumb side.

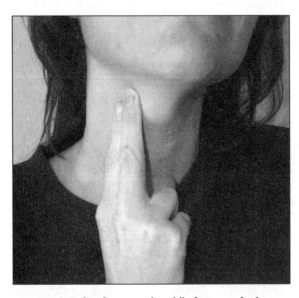

Use your index finger and middle finger to find your pulse on the side of your neck. Your pulse point is in the groove just on either side of the center of your neck.

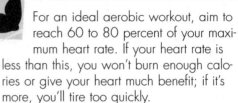

In the Mirror

For an ideal aerobic workout, aim to reach 60 to 80 percent of your maximum heart rate. If your heart rate is less than this, you won't burn enough calories or give your heart much benefit; if it's more, you'll tire too quickly.

Here's an example: Pamela is 53 and has a resting heart rate of 72 beats per minute. She subtracts her age from 220 (220 – 53 = 167). Next, she subtracts her 1-minute resting heart rate from 167 (167 – 72 = 95). She then multiplies 95 by 0.6 and 0.8 (95 × 0.6 = 57, 95 × 0.8 = 76). Finally, she adds her 1-minute resting heart rate to each of these results (57 + 72 = 129, 76 + 72 = 148). Her aerobic exercise heart rate training zone is 129 to 148 beats per minute. That means Pamela should exercise at an intensity that keeps her heart rate between 129 and 148 beats per minute.

This heart rate training zone is basically 60 to 80 percent of what your heart is capable of. Exercising below 60 percent still burns calories, but your heart won't see much benefit, and it will probably be so easy that you won't even know you're exercising. On the other hand, anything above 80 percent is too high. At this point, you start burning more carbohydrates instead of fat because you have to provide energy quickly to support the work you are doing, and fat is burned better at lower heart rates. Additionally, when you start exercising above 80 percent of your target heart rate, you won't be working out for long—you will get fatigued before you burn enough calories to make a difference.

So where in this heart rate training zone, ideally, should you aim for? There is obviously a difference between 60 percent and 80 percent. If you are a beginner, stay in the range of 60-65 percent until you become accustomed to your program, and move up from there. If you've been exercising a while, aim for the range of 70 to 75 percent and go from there. No matter where you start, eventually your fitness level will improve, and you'll need to increase your level of intensity.

When you get to the point that you finish a workout and don't really feel like you've worked that hard—you haven't really broken a sweat or feel like your muscles have had much of a workout—it's time to reach for a higher target heart rate. You should also intensify your workout if you aren't reaching your fat-loss goals and you feel that you can handle a tougher program. You'll burn more calories and get quicker results when you work at a higher heart rate. However, don't increase your exercise intensity before your body is ready. Jumping to the high end of the scale just to burn more calories isn't worth it if that exercise session wipes you out and makes you sore. Give your body a chance to get used to a certain level of intensity before you ratchet it up.

Spot Me

Don't push your body too hard. Let your body adjust to one exercise intensity before you go faster, higher, or farther.

You can check your heart rate during your workout in one of two ways: 1) you can manually check your pulse, or 2) you can use a personal heart-rate monitor. Manually checking your pulse is a bit cumbersome if you are bouncing up and down or moving around too much. I prefer to use a personal heart-rate monitor, which is a great tool to have. Heart-rate monitors have become very inexpensive ($25–$50) and are available at just about every sporting goods store or online. They provide you with instant readings, and some can be programmed to alert you if your heart rate gets too low or too high.

Calculate Your Rate of Perceived Exertion

The second means of determining the appropriate intensity of an aerobic workout is called a *rating of perceived exertion*, or *RPE*. Like a heart rate training zone, an RPE is individualized. It is a subjective measure of how hard you feel you are working.

Trainer Talk

The **rating of perceived exertion**, or **RPE**, is another means of figuring out the appropriate intensity of your aerobic workout based on how you feel during the workout. Shoot for a rating of between 5 and 6—moderate to somewhat hard—during your workout.

An RPE has a holistic approach to reaching your target intensity by combining all of the feelings you have during an exercise into one number. Your current RPE is a measure of how hard you feel you are working, taking into account how hard you are breathing, how your muscles feel, how much you are sweating or how hot you are, and how much more you think you can take. An RPE measure is made on a scale of 1 to 10; 1 is equivalent to absolutely no effort at all (lying down), and 10 is the highest level of exercise intensity you have ever felt. At an RPE of 10, you would feel that you're about to fall over: you can't go any further or any longer—it's the absolute max. Here's how the scale ratings break down:

1—Nothing at all
2—Extremely light
3—Very light
4—Light
5—Moderate

6—Somewhat hard

7—Hard

8—Very hard

9—Very, very hard

10—Absolute maximum

You should aim for a level of aerobic exercise that's equal to an RPE of 5 to 6 (moderate to somewhat hard). If you are being honest about your level of exertion, an RPE of 5 to 6 should also put you in your heart rate training zone. This makes RPE really cool: you don't have to monitor your heart rate when you get the hang of it; you'll just know that you are in the right zone based on how you feel. As you become more fit, you will increase the percentage of your heart rate that you train at, but the RPE should stay the same—the exercise will always feel moderate to somewhat hard. If your workout ever becomes "light," you know that you need to bump it up a notch.

Remember that a rating of perceived exertion is different for everyone. What may be moderate for you might be very hard for someone else. This is an individualized way of determining exercise intensity, but it's useful when you switch between forms of exercise. For instance, on a treadmill, you may feel moderate (RPE of 5) in your heart rate zone of 70 to 75 percent, but when you go jogging outside, you may feel moderate in your heart rate zone of 65 to 70 percent. All exercises are not created equal, so you will feel different with each one and have a different comfortable training zone with each one. Using an RPE measurement is a good way to equate different exercises. If you are always between a 5 and a 6 on the RPE rating, you know that you are within your training zone and are making progress toward your knockout look.

Machines, Classes, and the Great Outdoors

You can get the aerobic exercise you need in many ways, each beneficial in its own way. Nothing is magical about a treadmill or stair-stepper; nothing is life changing about riding a bike. These are just different ways of moving your body and working your heart, to help you burn calories.

So what type of aerobic exercise should you do? I say, do everything you can. Try every machine in the gym; get outside and do different activities when the weather's nice. Go beyond what your body is used to, and find new ways to shed extra pounds—while also having fun. Each type of aerobic exercise works different muscles in different ways. Some concentrate on the legs, some on the arms, and some put everything together to test your coordination as well. Here are some knockout options:

In the gym:

◆ Treadmills
◆ Stationary bikes
◆ Stair-steppers
◆ Ellipticals
◆ Cross-country ski machines
◆ Rowing machines
◆ Arm bikes
◆ Recumbent bikes
◆ Step-mills
◆ Aerobic classes

Outside:

◆ Walking or jogging
◆ Cycling
◆ Swimming
◆ Skating
◆ Rowing or kayaking
◆ Mountain biking
◆ Stair climbing

Start with the activities that you feel comfortable with and already enjoy. Any activity can become boring or tedious (which means that it will be harder to stick with for any length of time), so experiment with new gym equipment or outdoor activities to discover what you like or don't like. If you hate a certain machine, don't force yourself to use it. Choose an alternative, such as a group class or outdoor sport.

Science Sez

Research has shown that people who participate in a variety of activities stick with their exercise program longer and make more progress than people who do the same thing day after day. Mixing up your workout with different aerobic exercises makes your heart work at different levels and uses your muscles in different ways.

Another factor to consider when choosing your aerobic exercise is the number of calories it will burn. Exercises that make you support your own body weight and move more of your muscles (treadmill, aerobics class, skating) burn more calories than exercises done sitting down or using only some of your muscles (stationary bike, stair-steppers, ellipticals). If your goal is to lose extra fat, choose exercises that work as many of your muscles as possible (swimming, using a rowing machine or cross-country ski machine, jogging) so you can reach your goal faster. If you're maintaining your current fitness level, take advantage of less strenuous exercises that don't burn as many calories.

Machines for Every Movement

Personally, I think the treadmill is boring. I won't go near one—I'd rather walk outside. But that's me. I don't mind the weather, but some people hate the cold of winter and the heat of summer, and would rather walk inside with a nice fan blowing just the right amount of air on

them. I don't have any problem with that—as long as they are exercising, that's all that matters.

The benefit of indoor aerobic exercise is that there are so many options nowadays. I remember the days of having a choice of a treadmill, a bike, or a stair-climber. Now we have rowing machines, cross-country ski simulators, and even kayak simulators! You can participate in exercises that may not be available to you in the real world (when was the last time you went cross-country skiing during the summer?).

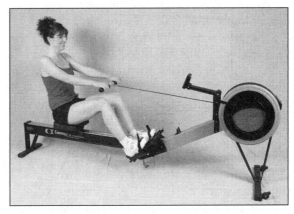

The rowing machine combines both your upper- and lower-body muscles for a full-body workout.

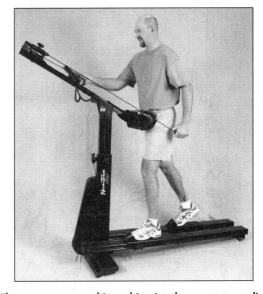

The cross-country ski machine involves some coordination and balance while getting your heart rate up.

Indoor aerobic machines have evolved to make exercise sessions more comfortable or more intense. You won't find as many of the old stationary bikes in the gym anymore. The reclined-position recumbent bike has grown in popularity because it is more comfortable and doesn't require you to hold on to it—just sit back and pedal. On the other hand, spin-bikes have taken the opposite approach and made the original stationary bike feel more like the bike you ride outside. A smaller seat and a more racinglike position really crank up the heart rate. Even the old stair-climbing machines have seen some improvements (and by improvements, I mean new ways of making it more intense). The stair-climbing machine has always been a great way to work on your legs and hips, but the newer climbing machines also give you the option of working your arms at the same time—more like climbing an endless ladder.

So working out inside doesn't have to be boring or tedious. Most gyms today have at least 5 to 6 different machines to choose from, and maybe as many as 10 to 12! As I mentioned earlier, the more different activities you can get your body involved in, the faster those knockout results will arrive—and the less chance you will quit because your exercise puts you to sleep.

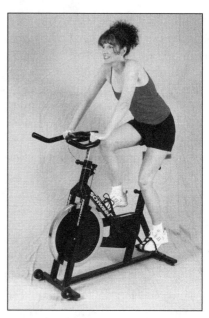

The spin bike puts your body into a racinglike position, which is more like riding a bike outside.

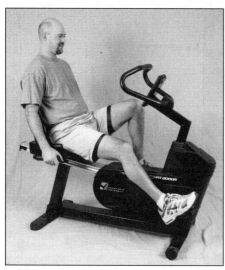

The recumbent bike is more comfortable and takes the stress off your arms so you can focus on your legs.

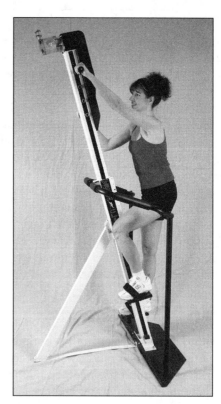

The full-body climbing machines get every muscle you have into the game.

Aerobic Classes

Since the early days of Jazzercise, aerobic classes have provided a fun way to get your heart rate up, burn calories, and have fun while working every muscle you have. Aerobic classes are different from other cardiovascular exercises because the movements are not repetitious (not the same thing over and over). You can take classes in regular floor aerobics, step aerobics, pump aerobics (which include weights), cardio-kickboxing aerobics, and several other varieties.

Aerobic classes teach you coordination and balance, and work another facet of fitness that we haven't talked about yet: the ability to make your body follow orders. The aerobics instructor usually doesn't tell you before class starts exactly what you are going to be doing, so you have to pay attention and get the message to your muscles as fast as possible. This makes aerobic classes kind of like an exercise for your brain as well. If your mind is not on what is happening, your body won't be following along with everyone else. This is a fun way to keep you engaged in the exercise, prevent boredom, and give your body all kinds of new stimulus to change.

Take It Outside

If you're like me, after being inside all day long, I'm ready for some fresh air. Thousands of people exercise outside every day either walking, jogging, riding their bike, or skating. I even count swimming in a pool as outdoor exercise because you aren't standing or sitting in one place—you're moving. Outdoor exercise engages the mind as well as the body. You have to move your body in response to your surroundings, moving in new ways and using your muscles in different patterns to produce a knockout look. This is a really cool point: moving outside is different from moving inside on a machine. Your muscles have to propel you

forward against the friction of the ground, maybe through a headwind, and around obstacles you won't find in a gym. All these things make your body work harder and differently than on a machine—which makes it a higher-intensity exercise. In fact, most of the time, exercise outside can be done at a lower speed (jogging at 4 miles per hour instead of 5 miles per hour on the treadmill, for instance), to keep your RPE in the right place.

Spot Me

If you are exercising outdoors, be aware of extreme temperatures (cold or hot). Your body may have trouble keeping warm enough outside on cold days, or it may get too hot during the summer months. The best time to exercise during the summer is early in the morning or in the evening. During the winter, the middle of the day is the warmest.

Which Comes First, Time or Intensity?

As you are putting together the aerobic part of your knockout workout, you will come to a point at which you have to make a decision: should you increase the amount of time you train, or how hard you're training in the time you have?

The answer to this question depends on which of three possible scenarios fits you best: 1) you aren't getting as much aerobic exercise as you'd like, but you just don't have any more time to give, 2) you are already exercising as long as you want to and don't want to go longer, or 3) you aren't getting as much as you want and probably have some room in your schedule to add more.

Intensity Before Time

If you are already squeezing in as much time as you can for aerobic exercise, and you don't have any more room in your schedule to add more, concentrate on increasing the intensity of your workout. This allows you to burn more calories in the time that you have already set aside. Consider adding more time only when you feel that you're working as hard as you can.

If you are already exercising as long as you want to, consider increasing your intensity as well. Sure, you might be able to add more time, but there comes a point at which too much exercise can stress your muscles and joints to the point of injury, plus delay your body's recovery time. So in these two scenarios, the rule is intensity before time.

Time Before Intensity

If you aren't at your time limit yet and do have room in your schedule to add more time, do it. When you reach your personal time limit, you can increase the intensity, but first put in as much aerobic training time as you can: it's always easier to go longer at a lower intensity than it is to go shorter at a higher intensity.

Cooling Down

The final part of your aerobic-training workout should always include a good cool-down. Far too often I see people get off the treadmill or bike, or come in from their jog, and go straight to their flexibility training—or, worse, go to the locker room and get dressed. Cooling down after you have your heart rate up is very important.

Your heart is a pump—it pushes blood out. Your heart cannot suck blood back to it. When you exercise, your heart pumps a lot of blood to your muscles, and when your muscles contract, they squeeze the blood back to the heart. When you suddenly stop moving, all the blood that has been sent to your muscles stays there—very little of it gets back to the heart. This causes your heart rate to increase even more, instead of slowing down, as it should after you exercise. This can lead to dizziness or lightheadedness, and in some cases, it can even cause a heart attack.

To cool down properly, spend time moving at a lower intensity until your heart rate returns to its resting level. If you've been jogging, cool down by walking. With cardio machines, reduce the intensity until your heart rate comes down. Walking is always a safe bet for a good cool-down.

The Least You Need to Know

◆ You can do many types of aerobic exercise—choose an activity or machine that you enjoy, and you'll be more likely to stick with it.

◆ To lose a pound, you need to burn 3,500 calories. To lose a pound per week, add activity that will burn an additional 500 calories per day.

◆ For aerobic activity, try to reach 60 to 80 percent of your heart rate reserve as you exercise.

◆ The longer and more intense your aerobic workout is, the more calories you'll burn.

◆ The rating of perceived exertion is a different way to measure the intensity of your workout and is beneficial for comparing one form of exercise to another.

◆ Always cool down after an aerobic workout—skipping it can make you feel dizzy or, worse, lead to a heart attack.

In This Chapter

- ◆ Fitness benefits without any sweat
- ◆ Basic rules of what, when, and how long to stretch
- ◆ Help your muscles feel better and relieve stress and tension
- ◆ Stretches for every part of your body

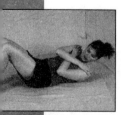 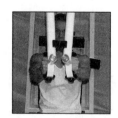 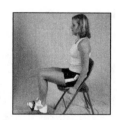 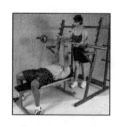 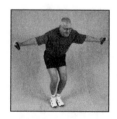 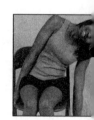

Chapter 6

Stretching It Out

As far back as I can remember, my college professors always told me how important stretching and flexibility training were in a complete fitness program. However, when it came time to tell us how to stretch, when to stretch, and what to stretch, the instruction became vague and generalized.

I have found the same situation in the popular fitness magazines and literature—just not enough info for you to make a good decision. It's not that there isn't enough information about flexibility—whole textbooks have been written on the subject. But the benefits of cardiovascular and strength training have overshadowed the benefits of flexibility so much that stretching has almost been pushed aside. It's time to fix that and make stretching just as important as any other part of your exercise routine.

Fitness Is Flexible

Just like breathing, stretching is something you do every day. When you get out of bed in the morning and raise your arms over your head and yawn really big, that's a stretch (and it feels good, doesn't it?). I think stretching has a bad rap partly because it can be painful if you do it incorrectly—which, unfortunately, is very common.

So why is *flexibility* important? Because the ability to move your body through its normal range of motion is part of being fit. What good is a strong heart and a good-looking body if you can't bend over to tie your shoes (don't laugh, it happens), can't sleep because your back hurts, or groan every time you try to get up off the couch. Flexibility is not about becoming a contortionist; it's about moving with ease, reducing muscle stress and strain, and feeling your muscles relax when you aren't using them. Flexibility is fitness. You can't be fit if you aren't flexible. You can look good without being flexible—just don't try to move.

Trainer Talk _____

Flexibility is defined as the ability to move through a full range of motion at a normal speed without any help.

Now, I need to dispel a couple of myths about stretching and stretching-related workouts. Stretching does not lengthen your muscles permanently. You cannot get longer, slimmer-looking muscles by stretching. I've often heard claims that exercise disciplines such as Yoga and Pilates lengthen your muscles and stretch your body into a different shape. That just can't happen. Muscles are connected to bones. For a muscle to be lengthened, it would have to be detached from a bone and reattached somewhere else farther down. The result would be an inability to move and a lot of pain!

Additionally, stretching will not keep you from getting sore after a workout. Soreness is a sign that your workout was a little too intense for you, and that some small level of damage was done within the muscle. Stretching doesn't fix that or make it feel any better. The key to not getting sore is not doing too much at one time, as we talked about in Chapter 3.

Stretching simply undoes the tension that is generated within a muscle when you contract it during a workout or movement. For instance, when you bend your elbow, you are shortening (contracting) the bicep muscle. When your elbow is straightened back out, the tension you generated doesn't disappear entirely—the muscle is still a little contracted. To release all the tension and totally relax a muscle, you have to stretch it beyond its normal resting length for a few seconds.

By now you're probably wondering how stretching and flexibility will help you build your knockout body. To be honest, flexibility won't show up in the mirror or be noticeable to anyone around you—but it will help you complete your knockout workouts easier because your body will move more fluidly and with less tension. Flexibility is sort of a helper to your workout—it provides the means for your muscles to do their job without getting too tight.

Science Sez _____

Flexibility training has never been proven to reduce the soreness that results from too hard of a workout. Stretching *can* help your body reduce normal everyday tension buildup.

Stretching the Rules

When I visit a gym and observe people who are stretching (or think they are stretching), I usually see more things being done wrong than right. I once had a student ask me, "If stretching is so easy, how can you do it wrong?" It was a good question. Any stretching is better than none, but a good-quality stretch is better than a simple lazy stretch. We can go through the moves of stretching without really adding to our flexibility—that's called a waste of time. When it comes time to train your flexibility, you have to be serious about it and do it right to get the most out of it. It isn't hard, and it isn't painful. In fact, if done right, it feels pretty darn good! But like I said before, general stretching guidelines don't really help. If you are like me, you want direct answers without any beating around the bush. So here's the truth.

What to Stretch

Every muscle that has been shortened or contracted during a workout needs to be stretched back out. This helps reduce muscular tension and relaxes a muscle quickly. If you do a set of bicep curls, you need to stretch your biceps. If you do a set of leg extensions, you need to stretch your quadriceps. If you move it, stretch it.

Likewise, the muscles that you didn't work out need to be stretched. Why? Because you want to *keep* your muscles flexible. When a muscle is stretched, it increases its level of flexibility. However, when you don't stretch, a muscle slowly tightens back up over time. Flexibility is not something that you just have. You have to work to keep it. Stretching muscles that you haven't worked ensures that they will remain flexible and ready for the next time you do work them out. It's a simple strategy to prepare your body to move later.

I could give you enough different stretches to fill another book, but I've picked just some of my favorites to show you in this chapter. These are the stretches that I feel you can get the most out of and that really make the muscles relax. You should work your way through each stretch for every muscle in this chapter to decide which ones you enjoy most and which ones feel the best to you. Some stretches pull on a muscle a little more than others. Depending on how flexible you are, a stretch may be easy or difficult for you, so try them all.

Deciding what muscles to stretch is easy:

◆ **Rule #1:** If you work it out, stretch it.

◆ **Rule #2:** If you don't work it out, stretch it.

◆ **Rule #3:** Your flexibility program should incorporate at least one stretch for each muscle group—about 10 stretches total.

When to Stretch

Since your muscles move all the time, even when you aren't working out, you can stretch at any time of the day or night (if you can't sleep, try stretching to relax your body). That being said, a warm muscle has more blood flow into and out of it, and has already been moving some, so it will stretch easier and more completely. A muscle that is cold (you haven't worked it yet) won't stretch as far or as easily. If you stretch before a workout or without warming up first, you won't be able to stretch as far— and you *shouldn't* try to stretch as far. I like to use the analogy of comparing your muscles to chewing gum. When gum is warm, it stretches easily and very far. When gum is cold, it doesn't stretch, but usually just breaks into pieces. Your muscles won't actually break into pieces, but research supports an increased chance of tearing a muscle if you stretch it too far when it's cold.

Spot Me _____

You can decrease your chance of pulling a muscle if you stretch it after you have warmed up or completed your exercise routine.

Follow these basic rules for when to stretch:

◆ **Rule #4:** The best time to stretch is when you have already worked out each muscle.

◆**Rule #5:** When you are stretching a muscle that hasn't been worked out or is cold, stretch more slowly and not as far.

How Long to Stretch

If you understand what you should stretch and when you should stretch, you can still mess it all up if you don't stretch long enough. This is probably the biggest mistake I see when I watch people go through their stretching routine. It's also why most stretching routines fail to perform. Research shows that stretching anywhere from 5 seconds to 2 minutes does some good, but there is an optimal time during which you get about as much increase in flexibility as you are going to get—that's at 30 seconds. If you hold each stretch for 30 seconds, your flexibility will increase quickly.

The hardest part of holding a stretch for 30 seconds is making sure that every second is a good-quality stretch. One of the neatest things our bodies do is let us know when we are pushing too far—usually by sending little pain signals to the brain. You never want to stretch until it hurts, but it should be a stretch. Knowing the difference is what makes a quality stretch work.

Think of it this way: when you are sitting still, you don't feel any stretch. When you start to pull the muscle beyond its normal resting length, you feel a stretch. If you stretch too far, it becomes painful. The goal is to get to that second part—when you have a sensation of stretching, but not one of pain. It may be a little uncomfortable, but not painful. If you hold that position when you have a sensation of being stretched, your body will slowly "turn off" the nerve endings that are sending the sensation to your brain. That's called *down regulation*. All of the sudden, it will feel like you aren't stretching anymore—that's the perfect place to be.

Trainer Talk

Down regulation is what happens when your nerve endings stop sending signals of stretch sensations to your brain.

Here are your rules for how long to stretch:

◆ **Rule #6:** Hold each stretch for 30 seconds—no more, no less.

◆ **Rule #7:** Hold each stretch at the point you can feel the sensation of being stretched, but don't make it painful.

A Simple Stretching Plan

Okay, now you know the rules of stretching, so all we have to do is find some good stretches and get to work. If you've done the math so far, you've figured out that if you do 10 stretches for 30 seconds each, you will spend about 5 minutes of your day stretching. That's not as bad as you thought it was going to be. Five minutes at the end of a workout is all it takes to train your body to be flexible, to reduce the tension your muscles generated during that workout, and to help your body move more fluidly. I can't make it any easier than that.

Now the fun part—the actual stretches. These *static* stretches are just a sampling of what I believe are the best stretches for each muscle group. You may find other stretches you like better, which is fine with me—as long as you actually do them. I suggest you go through each of these stretches, try them, and find which ones you like the best—that is, which ones produce the most stretch. Every now and then, you'll have to change the stretches you use so you don't get stuck doing a stretch that isn't really stretching you anymore.

Trainer Talk

The stretches you'll learn here are called **static** stretches because you move into a position and hold that position for 30 seconds. You are "static," or "not moving," during the stretch.

Abdominals

The abdominal muscles don't usually get very tight, even if you do a lot of ab exercises; but that doesn't mean you can ignore stretching them. Your abs work all the time in helping your back maintain good posture, so they deserve a break once in a while, and a good stretch really feels nice.

Inverted Superman

1. Lie down on your back on a carpeted surface or exercise mat.
2. Straighten your legs, point your toes away from you, and reach over your head with both arms.
3. Try to make your body as long as you can, pushing your toes away from you and your hands over your head.
4. It's okay to arch your back a little to get the biggest stretch possible. Your goal is to get to the point that you can lay your arms flat on the floor over your head (all the way from your shoulders to your hands).

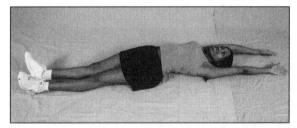

Inverted Superman stretch—make yourself as long as you can.

Twisted Cross

1. Lie on the floor on your back on a carpeted surface or exercise mat.
2. Bend your knees and slide your feet up until they are about a foot away from your butt.
3. Move your arms out to your sides, palms up and relaxed.
4. Breathe deeply as you roll your knees to one side. As you let them fall toward the floor, keep your feet together—this means one foot should leave the floor and rest on the bottom foot.
5. Press your knees toward the floor as far as you can—the goal is to lay your knees on the floor. Be sure to keep your shoulders down—if your upper body starts to roll over, stop and relax into the stretch right there.
6. Repeat this stretch on the other side.

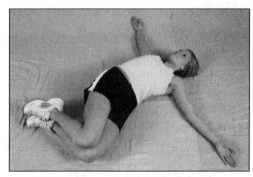

Twisted cross stretch to the left side.

Ball Arch

1. Lie across the top of a stability ball or big pillow so that it's in the middle of your back.
2. Stretch your legs away from you as far as possible, keeping your heels on the floor and pointing your toes toward the ceiling.
3. Reach over your head with both arms.
4. Let your back muscles relax while you reach back and down with your arms until you can touch the floor.
5. Your head and neck should be relaxed and will probably be lower than your chest, so keep breathing deeply throughout the stretch.

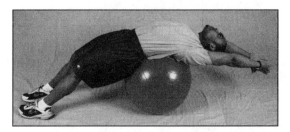

Ball arch stretch using a stability ball.

Chest

The muscles in your chest all attach to your upper arm and affect how your shoulders feel. When the chest is really tight, the shoulders roll forward, making you appear hunched over. Keep these muscles loose and flexible to maintain good posture and excellent range of motion.

Double Pull

1. Stand inside an open doorway (preferably one without a door) or next to an exercise machine, and hold on to each side at about elbow height.

2. Step forward until your arms are stretched out behind you.

3. Take one step back and then lean forward until your arms are stretched out again and the weight of your body is pulling you forward. Your chest and head should be in front of your feet at this time.

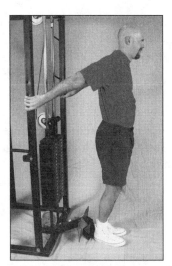

Double pull chest stretch.

Tabletop

1. Kneel on the floor in front of a chair, a stability ball, or anything that's about 2 feet high.

2. Place both hands on top of the chair, and scoot back until you are reaching forward to keep your hands on the chair.

3. Drop your head between your hands and push your shoulders toward the floor. Pretend you are trying to make your body into a tabletop from your hips to your hands (nice and flat).

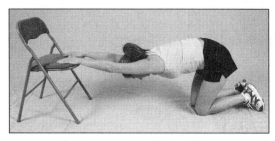

Tabletop stretch using a chair.

Lying Reach

1. Lie on your back on an exercise bench or stability ball.

2. Hold a 5- to 10-pound dumbbell in each hand. Hold your hands out to your sides, arms straight.

3. Let your arms fall toward the floor until you feel the stretch begin. Relax your chest and shoulders as much as possible.

4. When you are done, set down the dumbbells and relax.

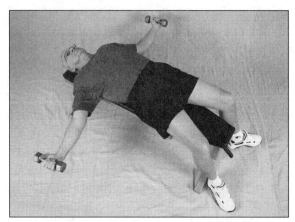

Lying reach stretch on an exercise bench.

Back

A bad back isn't just the fault of weak muscles. The muscles in the back can be overly tight and cause the same type of pains as a pulled or over-worked muscle. Because your back is responsible for holding most of your upper body weight up when you are standing, having a flexible back will ensure that you are able to move however you want and lift whatever you want.

Headrush

1. Sit in a chair or on a stability ball with your feet wide apart.
2. Lean forward and reach toward the ground between your feet (don't fall out of the chair).
3. Tuck your chin to your chest and relax your arms so you lean forward as far as possible.
4. If your hands touch the ground, don't hold yourself up. Let your elbows bend so you can go down farther.

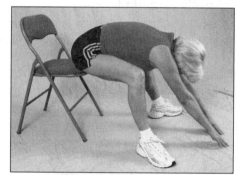
Headrush stretch for the lower back.

Pullback

1. Stand in front of an open door, pole, or exercise machine—basically, anything tall and strong enough that it won't move when you pull on it.
2. If you are using a door, grab hold of the doorknobs on each side. If you are using a pole or machine, grab hold about waist high.

3. Stand about 2 feet back, feet together, and lean back, pulling against the door or pole.
4. Let your arms relax until you start to feel the stretch in your upper back.

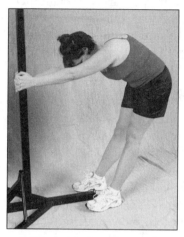
Pullback stretch using a pole.

Cat

1. Kneel on the floor on your hands and knees. Place your hands directly under your shoulders, and keep your knees directly under your hips. Keep your knees together and your hands shoulder width apart.
2. Lift your back in the air as far as you can. Pretend your spine is attached to a string that is being pulled up. Arch your back all the way from your shoulders to your hips.

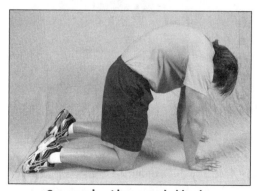
Cat stretch with a rounded back.

Shoulders

Ever try to move your arms without moving your shoulders? Bet you can't do it. So if you want to move your arms through their full range of motion, your shoulders better be flexible. Make sure to add some of these stretches to your plan to make that happen.

Turnaround

1. Stand facing a wall. Reach one hand out to your side (shoulder height), and place the palm of that hand against the wall.
2. Keep your hand against the wall while you turn your body away from that hand. If your right hand is against the wall, turn to your left, and vice versa.
3. Turn away until you really feel the stretch in your shoulder. Hold that stretch for 30 seconds, then repeat for the other arm.

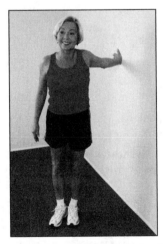

Turnaround stretch for the left shoulder.

Crosspull

1. Either sitting or standing, hold one arm straight out in front of you.
2. Use your other hand to grab hold of the elbow of the arm that is pointed out.
3. Pull this arm across your body until you feel the stretch in the back of your

shoulder. The arm being stretched should remain relaxed, while the arm pulling is doing all the work. Hold that stretch for 30 seconds, then switch to the other arm.

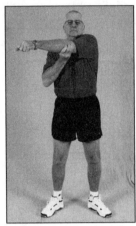

Crosspull stretch for the left arm.

Anchored Lean

1. Sit up nice and straight in a solid chair.
2. Reach down with one hand and grab hold of the bottom of the seat.
3. Keep a good grip on the seat while you lean your body toward the opposite side. This creates a stretch in the top of your shoulder and the side of your neck as that arm is being pulled.
4. Repeat this stretch on the other side.

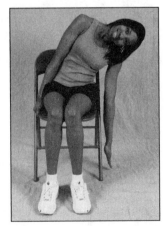

Anchored lean for the right shoulder.

Biceps

The biceps are probably the hardest muscle to stretch. I don't mean the hardest because they are tight, but because of the way they are attached in the body it's hard to really stretch out either end of the muscle. You won't feel much during these stretches, but make sure you do them to keep everything in balance.

Thumbs Down

1. Stand with your arms down to your sides, palms facing your thighs.
2. Make your hands into fists and point your thumbs out in front of you.
3. Lift both arms out behind you as far as you can. Your thumbs should now be pointed down. Hold this position while your biceps stretch. You won't feel a lot of stretch in this muscle, but it's happening.

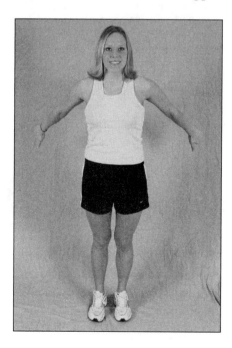

Thumbs down stretch for the biceps.

Twisters

1. Hold both arms straight out in front of you, hands open and fingers together.
2. Rotate your arms so your palms face down, and keep rotating in this direction until your palms face out to the sides and you start to feel the stretch.

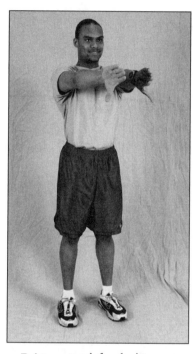

Twisters stretch for the biceps.

Triceps

For some reason I've always liked doing triceps stretches. Maybe it's because they really feel good, or that they are easy to do, or both. Whatever your reason, keeping these muscles loose really helps with biceps and back exercises that require the triceps to be flexible.

Back Scratch

1. Reach over your head with one hand like you are trying to scratch your back.
2. Use the other hand to reach up and pull on the elbow of the hand that is scratching your back.
3. Pull on the elbow until you feel the stretch in the back of that arm. Hold it for 30 seconds, then stretch the other arm.

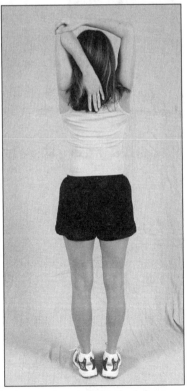

Back scratch stretch for the left triceps.

Reach Around

1. Reach over your head with one hand like you are trying to scratch your back.
2. Reach behind your back with the other hand and grab hold of the fingers on the hand that is reaching over your shoulder.
3. Pull down to create a stretch in the arm reaching over the shoulder. Hold this position for 30 seconds before switching positions and stretching the other arm.

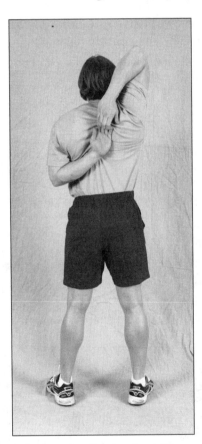

Reach around stretch for the right arm.

Hips and Butt

I know, I know—you are probably thinking "I want a tight butt, not a flexible one." You want the overall look of the muscle to be defined and not flabby, but you want the muscle to be able to move, so tightness is not a good thing in this context. A lot of the leg exercises you'll do will involve the hips and butt, so you'll want to include these stretches to keep yourself firm but flexible.

Diagonal

1. Lie on your back, legs straight and together, arms down at your sides.
2. Bring your right knee up toward your chest, and grab hold of that knee with your left hand.
3. You have to really let your leg relax now. Your left hand will hold your leg up. Relax your hips and leg, and let your foot drop so it hangs in the air.
4. Keeping your shoulders and hips on the floor, pull your knee across your body toward your left shoulder. If you aren't feeling the stretch, your leg isn't relaxed enough—there are muscles still tightened up. Let it all go!
5. Repeat on the other side by pulling the left leg across the body with your right hand.

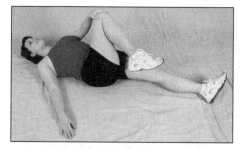

Diagonal stretch for the right hip.

Knee Squeeze

1. Lie on your back on the floor.
2. Bring both knees up toward your chest, and wrap your arms around your legs under your knees.

3. "Hug" your knees with your arms, pulling your knees toward your chest and squeezing until you feel the stretch in your hips and butt.

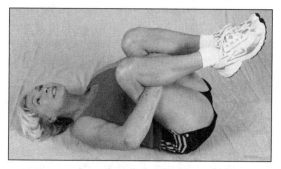

Knee squeeze stretch for the hips and butt.

Pretzel

1. Sit on the floor and place your legs straight out in front of you.
2. Bend one leg up and cross it over the other leg so that your foot is on the floor next to the other knee.
3. If your left foot is next to your right knee, place your right elbow on the outside of the left knee (the bent knee). Your other hand should be on the floor behind you supporting your upper body (see the picture for clarification).
4. Push against your knee to help twist your upper body and hips to the left as far as possible. Do not let your hips leave the floor.
5. Hold this position for 30 seconds and repeat on the other side.

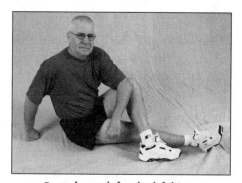

Pretzel stretch for the left hip.

Thighs

Nothing is worse than having thigh muscles that are so tight they hurt when you walk or climb stairs. There are a lot of nerve endings in these muscles that are activated when you stretch, meaning you will really feel this stretch.

Diamond

1. Sit on the floor. Bend your knees up toward your chest and keep your feet together.

2. Let your knees fall out to the sides so that your legs form a diamond shape (the four corners are the feet, knees, and groin).

3. Push down on each knee with your hands until you feel the stretch from the inside of your legs down toward your knees.

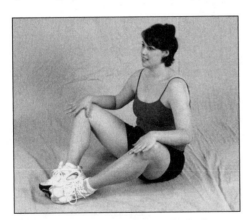

Diamond stretch for the inside thighs.

Quad Step

1. Place the toe of one foot on an exercise bench or chair. You may have to hold on to something for balance—that's fine.

2. Take a giant step out with the other foot.

3. Try to keep your torso as upright as possible while you push your hips down toward the floor. Your back knee may come in contact with the floor at the bottom.

4. If you don't feel the stretch in the front of your thighs, take a bigger step out. Hold the stretch for 30 seconds, then repeat on the other leg.

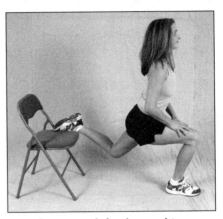

Quad step stretch for the quadriceps.

Side Skate

1. Stand with your feet together and your hands on your hips.

2. Take a big step out to one side. The leg that stays in place should stay straight, while the other leg bends at the knee.

3. Bend down as far as is needed to feel the stretch on the inside of the thigh on the leg that is straight. Hold this position for 30 seconds, then skate to the other side.

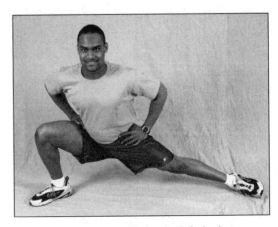

Side skate stretch for the left thigh.

Hamstrings

Nobody likes to stretch their hamstrings. Honestly, it doesn't feel that good, and it takes a long time to loosen them up. However, if you approach it slowly and keep at it, the ability to bend over without feeling any tightness in the back of your leg is well worth the effort.

Standing Toe Touch

1. Stand against a wall. Place your feet about a foot in front of you and about a foot apart.

2. Keep your hips against the wall as you slide your hands down the front of your legs until you start to feel the stretch in the back of your legs. The goal is to be able to touch your toes, but only go as far as you need to feel the stretch.

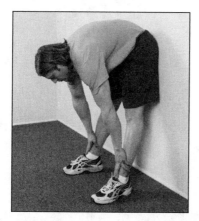

Standing toe touch stretch for the hamstrings.

Single Leg Reach

1. Sit on the floor.

2. Slide one leg straight so the toe is pointed up. Bend the other leg up close to the knee of the straight leg.

3. Reach out with both hands toward the toe of the straight leg. Reach until you feel the stretch in the back of that leg. The goal

is to reach your toes, but only go as far as you need to. Hold the stretch for 30 seconds, then switch legs.

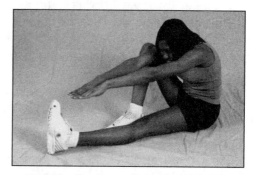

Single leg reach stretch for the left hamstring.

Lying Leg Pull

1. Lie on your back on the floor. Bend your knees up until your feet are about a foot from your butt.

2. Point one leg straight up in the air. Wrap a towel around your leg just below the knee or as close to the ankle as you can get. Hold on to the ends of the towel in both hands.

3. Pull on the towel, while keeping that leg straight, until you feel the stretch in the back of the leg. Hold the pull for 30 seconds, then change legs.

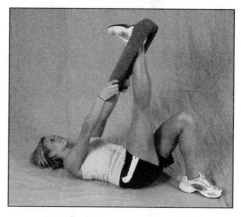

Lying leg pull for the right hamstring.

Calves

Calves are the easiest muscle to stretch, and you can stretch them just about anywhere—often without anyone knowing what you are doing. Keeping these muscles loose really helps your ankle flexibility and maintains a very sculpted look on your lower leg.

Wall Press

1. Stand facing a wall or doorway. Place the toe of one foot against a wall, and plant the heel of that foot firmly on the floor. The other foot should be behind you.

2. Lean forward so that your body weight pivots over the front foot until you start to feel the stretch along the back of your calf. Hold it for 30 seconds, then switch legs.

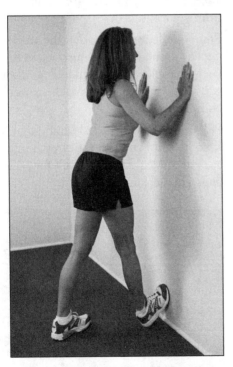

Wall press stretch for the right calf.

Curb Drops

1. Stand on a curb or the first step of a flight of stairs. You'll need to be able to hold on to something for balance.

2. Stand so that the balls of your feet are on the edge of the curb or step, and the rest of your feet are hanging out over the edge.

3. Relax your calves and let your body weight push your heels down toward the ground until you feel the stretch in both legs.

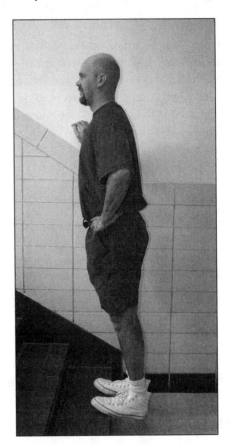

Curb drop stretch for calves.

In This Chapter

- ◆ What's in a calorie
- ◆ The lowdown on carbs, protein, and fat
- ◆ Dietary supplements
- ◆ Fill up with water
- ◆ A pyramid of food
- ◆ Ask a nutritional expert

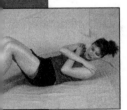
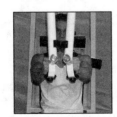
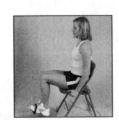
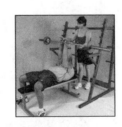
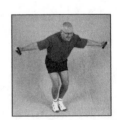
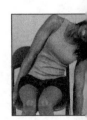

Chapter 7

Eating Exercises

"Sandy" was a client of mine for several years. For the first year or so, she hardly made any progress toward her goals, no matter how much I pushed her. I was beginning to think that she was somehow immune to exercise (also not a valid excuse). Then one day something happened. I was leaving the gym just after Sandy finished her workout. As I was driving out of the parking lot, I spotted Sandy's car pulling into a fast-food restaurant that just happens to specialize in ice cream. I pulled in and parked next to her and waited. When she came out, she was carrying a banana split—loaded with all the good stuff. I asked her what she was doing, and her reply was that I had told her she needed to eat immediately after a workout, to replenish her energy stores. She figured that right after getting a good sweat, it was the best time to eat the one thing she normally deprived herself of: lots of ice cream. She thought that her body needed all those calories and that she wouldn't have to feel guilty.

Do you see where I'm going with this? Turns out that the number of calories in that banana split was roughly equal to the number of calories she was burning during a workout. The moral to this story is that no matter how much exercise you do, a poor nutritional plan can sabotage your attempts at a knockout body. The food you eat is the fuel your body needs to build that new you, so it's worth a few pages to get the basics down.

Calories in and Calories Out

Exercise and nutrition are inseparable components of a knockout workout (and I'm not talking about how to work your jaw muscles). If you start thinking of food as fuel, it takes on a whole new meaning. Every *calorie* that you consume has to go somewhere. Some of it gets burned for energy; some of it may get stored to use later. In a perfect world, you would burn every calorie that you consumed, and you would consume just as many calories as you needed. To put this simply, it's just a matter of calories in versus calories out.

If your weight hasn't changed in a while, it's safe to say that you are burning just as many calories as you are consuming. If you have been gaining weight, you are probably eating more than you're burning off. And if you are losing weight, you are burning off more than you are eating. Piece of cake, isn't it? (Maybe I should say, slice of apple?)

> **Trainer Talk**
>
> A **calorie** is a unit of energy. No calories = no energy. That's why calories are absolutely necessary to provide the energy you need to maximize your knockout workout.

It seems that everyone is worried about calories—and probably rightly so. Advertisements for new foods often claim that they have fewer calories than other foods. Think about that—have you ever seen an ad claiming that a new and improved food has *more* calories than the regular food? Fact is, you can't live without calories because that's where we get our energy. You find calories in only three places: carbohydrates, fats, and proteins. Collectively, these are called nutrients because their calories provide energy. If a food doesn't fall into one of these categories, it doesn't have any calories. So if some newfangled diet food is supposed to be calorie free, you can bet that it doesn't have any carbohydrates, fats, or proteins (which should make you wonder what you are really ingesting). Things such as water, vitamins, herbs, spices, chemicals, and prescription drugs don't contain any calories because they aren't made of nutrients.

Any calorie-free food or drink is also energy free. I'm sure you've seen products that are supposed to boost your energy. But without any carbs, fat, or proteins, they can't do that—there is no source of energy. These products are usually full of chemicals and "natural" ingredients that may help the body in other ways we don't know about yet, but they don't provide energy.

Fill 'Er Up

To build that knockout body, you need the right fuel—and the right amount of fuel. Think of your body as a high-performance race car. If you put cheap fuel in a race car, it won't win any races. If you give your car the highest-octane fuel available, it will run like a champ. Your body works the same way. Food is your fuel, so if you give your body what it needs to run well, you will race toward that knockout look. If you feed it the wrong fuel, you'll just feel knocked out.

Carbohydrates

Carbohydrates should be the mainstay of your knockout nutrition. The carbohydrate is the primary fuel source the body uses during high-intensity activity such as resistance training—plus, the brain and nervous system use it almost exclusively for energy. Carbs have been getting a bad name lately, with all kinds of low-carb diets claiming that carbs make you fat. If you've noticed, those low-carb diets didn't make everyone skinny, and they were never endorsed by the experts of nutrition (the American Dietetics Association). You should actually feel good about eating carbohydrates because they are the "flame" that burns fat. The chemical processes in your body that turn food into energy need carbohydrates to work—especially when you need to process fat. When you run out of carbs—you *"hit the wall"*—your body has to rely on protein to help burn fat; this is a really slow process that decreases your energy levels and diminishes your ability to exercise.

Trainer Talk

"Hitting the wall" is a term that fitness enthusiasts use to describe the sensation of running out of carbs for energy. It feels like you actually ran into a wall—your body slows down, you have trouble thinking straight, and there is no way you can go on until you refuel. The only way to avoid this is to keep your body fed with carbohydrates.

Carbohydrates are usually categorized as either starches or sugars, which are actually quite different. Starches, also called complex carbohydrates, are found in whole grains, cereals, vegetables, and dried beans and peas. Sugars are broken down into two more categories: simple and refined. Simple sugars are found naturally in milk products and fruit. Refined sugars are manufactured and added to the foods you eat, usually in the form of sucrose and high-fructose corn syrup. Refined sugars make up a large part of sodas, fruit drinks, cookies, jam, candy, and ice cream. This is probably why carbohydrates have gotten a bad rap. If you eat a lot of foods with refined sugars, chances are, you'll gain weight because you end up eating a lot of calories that you don't burn off.

Unfortunately, the refined sugars taste good! This doesn't mean that you shouldn't ever eat products with refined sugars. If you tried to exclude refined sugars from your diet completely, you would probably find yourself eliminating some of your favorite foods (especially the sweet stuff). Instead, you should try to eat more of the complex "starch" carbohydrates whenever possible and save the refined sugars for special occasions and treats.

The starches (complex carbs) are the foods that our society has been eating less of but needs to eat more of. Few people eat fruits and vegetables every day, foods that contain complex carbs. In fact, a recent study of working adults found that the average person eats about half the amount of starches and twice the amount of refined sugars that they should.

So how many carbohydrates do you need? It depends. Most recommendations state that 55 to 70 percent of your total daily calories should come from carbohydrates, and that the majority of those should be from complex carbs (starches). It's pretty tough to have the same percentage of foods every day, so the range allows you to have some days when you have more carbs, and some days when you have fewer. You should try and get between 2.5 to 4.5 grams of carbohydrate for each pound you currently weigh. (Note that the number of carbs you need decreases if you lose weight.) This number represents enough carbs to support your workouts without having extra that can be stored as fat. For example, a 135-pound person needs to eat between 338 and 608 grams of carbs each day. On days when your activity level is higher, you should eat more carbs; on days when you don't exercise as much or are taking a day off, aim for the lower end of the range.

Proteins

Proteins are called the building blocks of the body because they are essential for muscle growth and keep all the body's systems working properly. However, high-protein diets do not make the body build muscle faster. Just as with carbohydrates, there is an optimal level of protein that your body needs; any extra will be stored as fat.

Protein is found in almost every type of food you can imagine. However, some foods, such as meats and eggs, are higher in protein. Other foods, such as fruits, don't have much protein. Unfortunately, some of the foods that are good sources of protein often have a large amount of fat. Good sources of protein include red meat, chicken, fish, eggs, beans, and legumes.

Protein is used for energy only if you have totally run out of carbohydrates. As I mentioned earlier, when you start to rely on the calories from protein for energy, your body slows down. It takes a long time to turn protein calories into the type of energy your muscles need (you actually turn them into a form of carbohydrate), and that causes your body to slow down. Another reason you don't want to rely on protein for energy is that if your body has to burn protein for energy, it can't use it to build muscle tissue. One of the goals of resistance training is to increase lean muscle tissue, so you want to make sure that the protein you eat is being used for that purpose, not for getting you through your workouts. After all, what's the point in exercising if your body doesn't have the protein you need to build muscle tissue? You basically end up spinning your wheels and exercising for nothing.

Because your protein calories mainly will be used for building lean tissue, you don't need a whole lot every day. Your protein intake should be between 12 and 15 percent of your total daily calories. This equals about 0.5 to 1 gram of protein for each pound you weigh. Our 135-pound person, therefore, needs 68 to 135 grams of protein each day. How much protein you eat each day does not depend on your activity level the way carbohydrates do. You should try to eat the same amount of protein every day because your body is always working on building lean muscle tissue if you are exercising on a regular basis. During the times you aren't exercising (while you work, sleep, watch TV, read this book) your muscles are recovering, which is when protein is needed the most. Strive to maintain adequate protein intake every day.

In the Mirror

Calculate your protein needs by multiplying your body weight by 0.5 and by 1. This is the range of grams of protein you should consume every day.

Fat

Before we start, you should note that not all fat is bad. Everyone requires some fat to keep the body working properly and aid tasks such as vitamin absorption and hormone formation. The problem is that the typical American diet is 34 percent fat, which is much too high. Both the American Heart Association and the Subcommittee on Nutrition of the United Nations agree that fat should provide between 15 and 20 percent of your daily calories. For most people, decreasing fat intake from just 34 percent to 20 percent will cause a reduction in body fat because the body will stop storing the excess. On the other hand, intakes of less than 10 percent have been shown to decrease testosterone production and muscle development, and decrease the body's ability to absorb vitamins A, D, E, and K. Even if you have some excess fat stored that you want to get rid of, you need to have fat in your diet. This is because your stored fat cannot help your body with vitamin absorption and other necessary processes. Only fat that is moving through the digestive process and through the bloodstream can do this.

Science Sez

You body requires fat to keep everything working normally. Without fat, you would not be able to absorb vitamins A, D, E, or K; and several chemical processes that help keep you alive would seriously slow down. Aim at eating 15 to 20 percent of your daily calories from fat. This will provide you with the fat your body needs without excess that your body will store as extra weight.

Here's the big news (make sure you remember this part): each gram of fat has more than twice as many calories as a gram of carbohydrate or protein (9 calories in fat versus 4 in carbs and protein). With so many calories in each gram of fat, you don't have to eat much fat to get 15 to 20 percent of your calories. Unfortunately, the things we love to eat (because they taste so good) usually have a lot of fat grams and, therefore, a lot of calorioes in them. Nature's cruel trick is that fat provides much of food's flavor and texture.

The final reason fat is important is that it does provide a lot of calories and is thus a great source of energy. However, this doesn't mean that you should eat more fat when you need more energy. You already have fat stored in your body that needs to be burned, so don't eat any more than you need (15 to 20 percent of your daily calories).

On Top of That

Dietary supplements line grocery store shelves, are touted in advertisements in your favorite magazines and newspapers, and now appear in specialty stores that only sell supplements. The key to keep in mind about dietary supplements is that they are what they claim to be: supplements. The word *supplement* means "in addition to." Supplements should never take the place of the carbohydrates, protein, and fat you get from regular food. However, they can help you get enough nutrients on days when you are extra busy, need a quick good-for-you snack, or are traveling and cannot cook for yourself.

Supplement manufacturers would have you believe that you can't possibly build a knockout body with regular food and that their product has something special that will make your nutrition better than that of your normal food-eating friends. These claims couldn't be further from the truth. Supplements can help you reach your goals, but they can't do it by themselves. Food is always your best fuel, but if you find that you are having problems getting enough food to meet the demands of your knockout workout, supplements can help.

That being said, the most helpful dietary supplements are those that provide calories in proportion to your regular eating habits. If you are trying to maintain a diet of 70 percent carbs,

15 percent fat, and 15 percent protein, look for calorie supplements that have about the same proportions. Most of the time, the serving size of a supplement will be close to that of a small meal or a large snack. These "meal replacements," as they are usually called, can provide you with good sources of nutrients and some of the vitamins and minerals you need. Examples are Slimfast shakes, SuperShake, Ensure, and even Carnation Instant Breakfast Drink. Even though the commercials say it's okay to "have one for breakfast, one for lunch, then eat a sensible dinner," you shouldn't rely on supplements because they do not have all the qualities of regular food: qualities such as taste, variety, texture … and taste. (Yes, I said *taste* twice.)

Besides drink form, supplements are often found as "energy bars" or "meal bars." Like their liquid counterparts, these are good for a little something extra but should not be regularly substituted for normal food. This is because supplements do not provide all of the necessary naturally occurring vitamins and minerals that foods do. Anything in a supplement has been chemically made, altered, or enhanced, which is not always a good thing.

Have a Drink

Have you ever sat down to a meal without something to drink? Probably not. Entire aisles in grocery stores are devoted to beverages of some form. Whether it's plain old water, milk, sodas, fruit juices, or even alcoholic drinks, there are tons of options to quench your thirst. The downside to this plethora of fluids is that you have to make another decision: what should you be drinking?

The human body consists of more than 75 percent water. Your muscles are mostly water, and even your fat has water. Clearly, water is extremely important. Does this mean that you should drink only plain water?

Thankfully, no, it doesn't. The main ingredient in all drinks is water, so no matter what you drink, you'll be getting the benefits of water. That said, it's important to note that plain old water is still the best thing for your body simply because many of the other choices have chemicals that we can't pronounce—and some can actually cause dehydration. There are several new choices on the shelves today that simply add some sort of flavor to water—grape water, orange raspberry water, citrus melon tropical water, and so on. If they don't have any calories, they are simply water with harmless chemical flavoring.

Fluids should serve one main purpose: to keep you hydrated. During hot and humid days, water is essential for survival. When you are in the middle of your knockout workout and get thirsty, water will quench that thirst faster than anything on the market. Sports drinks such as Gatorade and Powerade also help to quench your thirst and will provide you with replacement electrolytes and extra energy, but water has always been shown to be the most effective fluid for preventing dehydration.

If you do choose to use sports drinks, soda, or any other fluid with additional calories, be sure to account for these in your daily nutrition. I have seen numerous clients cut many calories simply by eliminating sodas, which can have as many as 150 calories per 12-ounce serving. Diet sodas are usually low calorie or calorie free, so they are basically just flavored water.

Eat Like an Egyptian

No this isn't a new *fad diet*, but an old friend known as the Food Guide Pyramid. I doubt the Egyptians had anything to do with this pyramid because you are actually the one who will be building it. Just like carbohydrates, the pyramid has taken its fair share of abuse over the years, but like the Energizer Bunny, it just keeps on coming back stronger than ever.

In 2005, the FDA unveiled the new pyramid based on the Dietary Guidelines for Americans that it developed with the help of hundreds of

nutrition experts. Of all the diet plans out there, this is the only one that doesn't go away and come back in a new wrapper every few years. In fact, this is the only nutritional plan that actually has tons of research to support it. The key is that it isn't the same for everybody (does that sound familiar to you?). Just like your knockout workout, your nutrition plan has to be tailored just for you, and the Food Guide Pyramid does just that. It's beyond the scope of this book to get into all the details of the pyramid simply because it has to be individualized just for you. This is a simple thing to do, so I encourage you to check out all the details at www.mypyramid.gov.

> **Trainer Talk**
>
> **Fad diets** get their name because they come on strong and fade fast, and then get recycled every few years. They never work for more than a few weeks, and they always require you to eat specific foods or give up specific foods.

Unlike most fad diets that try to keep you from eating certain foods or that force-feed you quantities of foods you never thought you would eat, much less like, the pyramid doesn't exclude anything. Everything is eaten in moderation, with guidelines on how much of certain food groups you should have. The different food groups include grains, vegetables, fruits, oils, dairy, and meats. Every food fits in the pyramid somewhere. The alternative is to try a diet that requires you to give up something (usually your favorite food). Can you guess what happens next? You crave that one food until you can't stand it anymore, and then you go out and eat way too much of it, making yourself sick. Sound familiar?

The Food Guide Pyramid gives you recommendations based on your age, gender, and how much exercise you get every day. Here's an example. For a 35-year-old female who exercises between 30 and 60 minutes every day, here is what it recommends for a daily nutrition plan:

- Eat around 2,000 calories every day
- At least 6 ounces of whole grains, preferably from at least 3 different food sources (breads, cereals, etc.)
- 2 $\frac{1}{2}$ cups of vegetables
- 2 cups of fruit
- 3 cups of milk products (low fat and calcium rich)
- 5 $\frac{1}{2}$ ounces of meat and beans

Fad diets come and go over and over again. Every few years there is a "new" diet that is exactly like one from about five years ago, just with a different name. If any of these actually worked for the long term, we would all be doing it, we'd all be knockouts, and the diet and fitness industry would be out of business. This obviously hasn't happened yet; don't hold your breath expecting the miracle diet to arrive next week.

Eating to fuel your body is as simple as following some simple rules and sticking to them all the time. Rule no. 1 is, don't deprive yourself of anything. Rule no. 2 is, don't binge on any one thing. Rule no. 3 is, eat a variety of foods from all the food groups. That's as simple as it can be. Maybe it's not easy in the beginning, but it's simple.

Ask an Expert

A fully developed nutrition program is beyond the scope of this book. Many good nutrition books are available (see Appendix B for a few I recommend) that can help you further in this area. The one thing that you need to realize when you are working on your eating habits is that you will never get them perfect. If you try to be perfect, you will fail. If you allow yourself the occasional slip-up, you can recognize the mistake, correct it, and get back to work. Additionally, nutrition is an ongoing process. As your body's needs change, so does how you fuel it. Proper dietary habits take time, don't happen overnight, and should be adaptable.

The best advice I can give you here is to seek the advice of a nutritional expert. Be aware that only licensed and registered dieticians are experts. Anyone who calls him- or herself a "nutritionist" is probably just someone who read a few books and knows how to decipher a food label. A dietician went to school, takes continuing education, and specializes in nutritional counseling. This is the kind of person you want to talk to.

The Least You Need to Know

- A calorie is simply a unit of energy; your body needs calories to keep functioning.
- Carbohydrates are not the enemy. Neither are proteins or fats. Taken in the right balance, the body needs all of them to function normally.
- Dietary supplements are meant to be an addition to your regular foods, not a replacement for them.
- Don't forget to hydrate your body! Water is the best hydrator, but sport drinks are also an efficient way to replace much-need fluids while pursuing your body-sculpting goals.
- The Food Guide Pyramid (www.mypyramid.com) is a great tool to help you design a nutrition program.
- Registered dieticians can analyze your eating habits and help you find ways to improve your nutrition.

In This Part

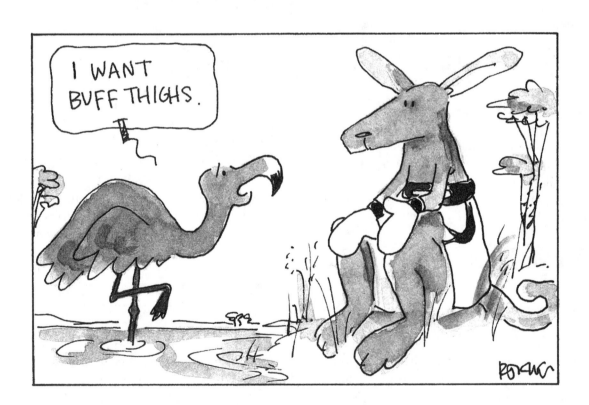

Part 3

Putting Your Muscles to Work

Proper tools help the mechanic keep your car running fine. When it comes to your body, exercise is the tool. The next 10 chapters provide all the tools you'll need to build that knockout body and keep it tuned up for a high-performance life. Each chapter focuses on a different muscle group or part of your body so that you can quickly find the exercises that will meet your needs and fit into your exercise plan. As you flip through these pages, you'll see that this is no normal exercise book filled with models—these are actual people who have learned how to do these exercises. I'm sure you've heard that exercise should be a part of everybody's life, not just those already in shape. For that reason, I've made sure that each exercise listed here includes instructions on how to modify it to fit you perfectly, whether you're 14 or 94. I also know that not everyone has a complete gym at their disposal, so some exercises can be done without big gym equipment—and some can be done without any accessories. Whether you want the basic model to get you from A to B, or the top-of-the-line model with all the bells and whistles, you'll find exercises in here for you.

In This Chapter

◆ Cheap alternatives to infomercial machines

◆ Exercises done lying down

◆ Crunching, twisting, and rolling your abs

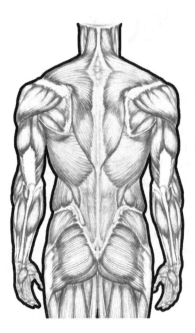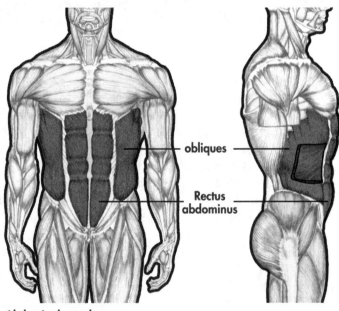

obliques

Rectus
abdominus

Abdominal muscles.

Chapter 8

The ABCs of Abdominals

Of all the parts of your body, the abdominals have been given the lion's share of attention over the last 20 years. I can't remember a time when there wasn't a new and improved abdominal exercise machine being touted on the late-night infomercials. What's really interesting is that those infomercials keep bringing back the same equipment every four to five years, as if we forgot we already bought it and then tossed it out when it didn't work as advertised. Those infomercials won't go away until we stop buying all that junk (and by junk, I mean trash).

The whole abdominal machine infomercial industry is fed by our unwillingness to just get down and do some old-fashioned exercises that we know work. What's really funny is that the exercises in this chapter are probably easier than any of those weird machines—and they actually work. I don't have an infomercial with flashy models and an easy payment plan, but I do have stacks of research that always comes to the same conclusion—the basic abdominal exercises always get the job done. Keep reading to find out how to avoid those three easy payments of $19.95. (See Chapter 3 for guidance on how many reps and sets to do, and an explanation of the levels assigned to the exercises in this and the following chapters.)

Crunches: Level 1

I recently did a poll of people who work out at the same gym I do. I asked everyone to name their favorite abdominal exercise. The overwhelming response was the crunch. I then asked them if that was really their favorite exercise, to which they usually responded with something like, "Well, I don't *really* like the crunch, but it's the most popular ab exercise." This is the sad plight of the crunch; it's a great exercise that doesn't get much love.

The crunch specifically targets the abdominal muscles, which are responsible for flexing your spine (probably the smallest exercise movement you will do), so they are a great isolation exercise. The crunch has a lot of variations, but they aren't all the same. Other exercises in this chapter have a similar look, but they work a little differently. It's a good idea to always start with the basic crunch before moving on to some of the more complicated variations.

Preparation

1. Lie on your back on an exercise mat or a carpeted surface. You can also do these on top of an exercise bench.

2. Bend your knees so that your feet are about 12 to 18 inches from your behind. Cross your arms over your chest so your hands touch your shoulders.

Spot Me _____

Don't hold on to the sides of your head, or put your hands under your head. You'll end up putting pressure on your neck when your abdominals get tired, which can possibly injure your neck.

Movement

3. Take a deep breath in. When you start to exhale, tuck your chin to your chest and roll your head and shoulders up off the floor. Stop when your shoulder blades leave the floor.

4. Breathe back in on your way down, slowly lowering yourself to the floor. Immediately start another repetition (no rest between these reps). Keep going until you've finished your set.

Variations

Level 2: Perform the same movement, but take away your base of support by lifting your feet off the ground. Now the challenge is in doing the crunch without rolling over sideways. For more fun, point your feet straight up in the air while you crunch.

Level 3: For even more resistance, hold a dumbbell or weight in the air over your head while you crunch with your feet pointed straight up. Focus on pushing the weight toward your feet with each repetition. Always remember to breathe with each repetition, but don't go so fast that you hyperventilate.

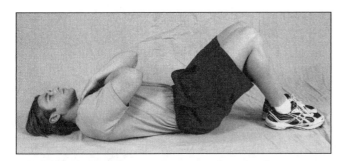

Crunch beginning and ending position.

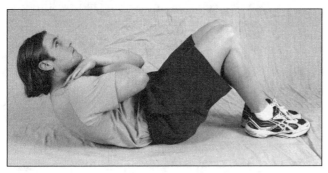

Crunch midpoint position—start breathing in.

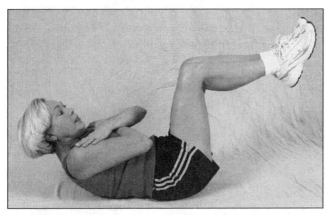

Crunch without your feet as a base of support.

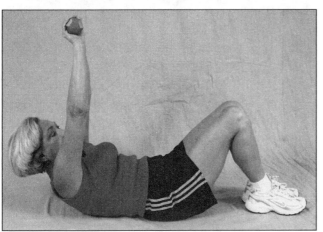

Crunch while holding a weight.

Oblique Crunches: Level 2

Pronounced *oh-bleak*, the oblique muscles are responsible for helping you rotate your torso from side to side. They also assist the big abdominal muscles during the sit-up and regular crunch. Without the oblique muscles, you wouldn't be able to turn around without moving your entire body from head to toe (which would make you look like Frankenstein). Since I'm sure you don't want that style of physique, the oblique crunch challenges your abdominals to a combination of rolling up and twisting at the same time.

Spot Me

If you've had any back problems, talk with your physician before starting this exercise. Oblique crunches aren't dangerous, but they do involve some twisting of your spine, so play it safe.

Preparation

1. Lie on your back on either a carpeted surface or an exercise mat (the hard floor isn't much fun). Bend your knees so that your feet are about 12 to 18 inches from your butt.

2. Reach up with both hands and touch your fingers to the top of your sternum bone just at the base of your neck. Don't push in—just rest your fingers there on the bone. Keep your elbows at your sides.

Movement

3. Take a deep breath in. As you exhale, lift one shoulder off the floor and roll up toward the opposite knee in a twisting motion. If you lift your left shoulder, aim toward your right knee (and vice versa). Your opposite shoulder, the one still on the floor, will want to roll up, too, so you have to concentrate on rotating and twisting to one side while you lift. Sometimes it helps if you pretend you are trying to see what's on the floor next to you.

4. Twist and roll up until the shoulder that's still on the ground can't stay there anymore and starts to come up. Slowly breathe in and let yourself back down to the floor.

5. Now do an oblique crunch to the other side, alternating left and right. One crunch to the right and one to the left equals one total repetition. Concentrate on keeping your hips from rolling left and right—this should all be happening in your trunk and shoulders.

Variations

Level 2: Of course, we can make this more challenging. Instead of alternating left and right, do an entire set on one side. This eliminates the brief period of rest the muscles get between repetitions.

Level 2: Take away your base of support by lifting your feet about 2 to 3 inches off the floor, for a greater challenge.

Level 3: If you want even more difficulty, try the bicycling oblique crunch: bring the opposite knee up toward your shoulder as you crunch (right shoulder and left knee, then left shoulder and right knee).

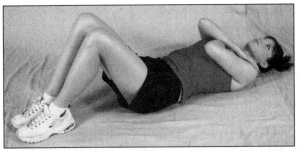

Oblique crunch beginning and ending position.

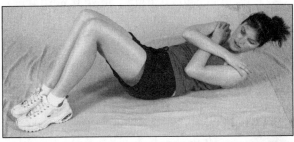

Oblique crunch midpoint position, left side.

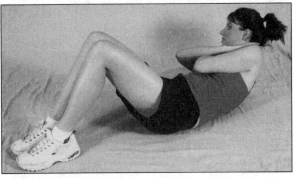

Obliques crunch midpoint position, right side.

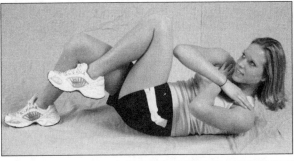

Bicycling oblique crunch to the left side.

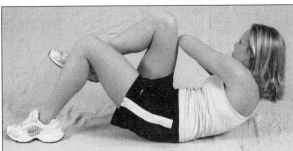

Bicycling oblique crunch to the right side.

Burner Abs: Level 1

You can feel some muscles the moment you start working. The abdominals fit into this category. You'll feel this great "burning" sensation when you really start to make the muscles work. Don't worry—you aren't on fire and nothing's wrong. In fact, everything is exactly right. Burner abs are all about making this sensation occur quickly and then holding it there for a long time. I know, it sounds painful, but it's not. The brain is releasing all those fun endorphins that make this sensation feel really good. The key to burner abs is speed and endurance. You'll do more reps in this exercise than just about any other exercise in this book. The speed component is important because although you're doing more of them, you're actually finishing each set faster than with any other abdominal exercise. Give it a try—you'll like it.

Preparation

1. Lie on the floor on your back. It's a good idea to double up your exercise mat, or use an exercise mat on top of your carpet. You can use a towel if you don't have a second mat. The extra cushion helps the movement of the hips during the exercise.

2. Cross your arms over your chest, placing your fingers on your shoulders.

3. Make sure your feet are 12 to 18 inches from your butt. It may also help to have someone hold your feet or to anchor them under something heavy, such as a couch.

Movement

4. Start with the first half of a basic crunch. Take a deep breath in, exhale, and lift your head and shoulders off the floor while keeping your chin tucked to your chest.

5. Don't go back down. While you hold your shoulders off the floor, twist your body so that one shoulder goes down toward the floor and the other points toward the ceiling. The more you can rotate your torso, the better. Don't let your shoulder touch the floor.

6. As soon as you have rotated as far as you can one direction, rotate the other direction. Now start doing this as fast as you can—all the while holding yourself off the floor.

7. This set is over when you can't stand it anymore, or you start getting sloppy or start slowing down. This exercise is all about speed, so keep it moving fast.

Variations

Level 2: Okay, I understand that this is already pretty taxing, but I can make it even more so. Instead of holding your feet to the floor, hold them up in the air with your legs pointed straight out away from you. Now you have to twist back and forth while balancing on just your hips and lower back—that's what the extra mat or towel is for. If you want even more challenge, lift your legs higher in the air.

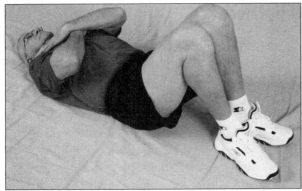

Burner abs beginning and ending position.

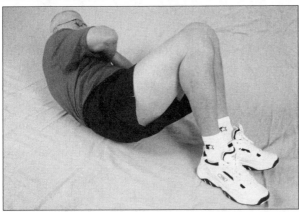

Burner abs midpoint position, twisting to the left.

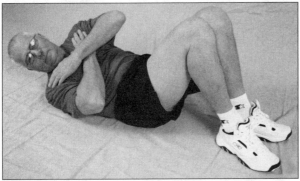

Burner abs midpoint position, twisting to the right.

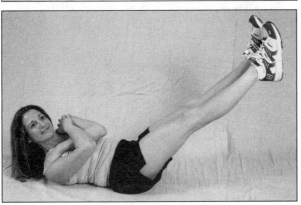

Burner abs with the legs straight out.

Sit-Ups: Level 2

If I were a betting man, I'd bet that sit-ups are one of the oldest known exercises. If you think about it, you do one every day when you wake up and "sit up" in bed—so why not do a few more? The sit-up has been given a bad rap the last few years, with a myth floating around that this exercise can hurt your back or that it isn't good for your abdominals. I'll say this only once: that's a total bunch of made-up phooey designed to get you to buy some crazy machine. The sit-up has always been a staple exercise for every athlete and fitness buff. The great thing about this exercise is that it doesn't work just the abdominals; it also works the muscles in your neck that control part of your head movements, and the muscles in your hips that help you walk. It isn't a head-to-toe exercise, but it is a head-to-hip exercise (and that's half your body).

Preparation

1. Lie down on the floor on a carpeted surface or an exercise mat. If you have trouble getting up and down off the floor, you can also do these while lying on an exercise bench or even on your bed (which makes them a great way to start your day).

2. Cross your arms over your chest, and touch your fingers to your shoulders.

3. Bend your knees so that your feet are about 12 to 18 inches from your butt. In the beginning, you'll need to anchor your feet under something heavy, such as a couch or bed, or have a workout partner hold your feet for you (later you'll be able to do this without an anchor).

Movement

4. Take a deep breath in. Tuck your chin to your chest and, as you exhale, slowly roll your head and shoulders off the floor.

5. When your shoulders are up, continue to lift your entire upper body off the floor until you can touch your elbows to your knees. You'll be doing a lot of pulling with the muscles in the top of your legs, known as the hip flexors, but keep those abdominals tight by thinking about flexing them.

6. Slowly breathe in and lower yourself back to the floor. Don't drop back to the floor as if you're done—going down is the last half of the exercise.

7. Take a deep breath and start another repetition. Keep repeating until you have finished your set.

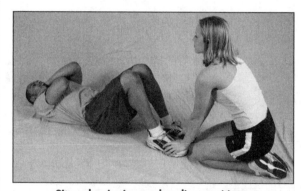

Sit-up beginning and ending position.

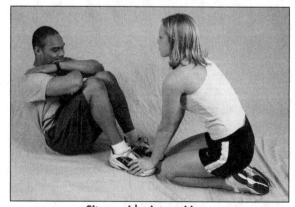

Sit-up midpoint position.

Variations

Level 3: Since the only weight you are lifting is your upper-body weight, sooner or later sit-ups will get easy. You can add more resistance by holding a weight against your chest. Use a small dumbbell, weight plate, or medicine ball of 5 to 15 pounds, depending on how much more resistance you can handle (always start small). If you need even more resistance, hold the extra weight over your head and finish your sit-ups at the position where your arms are pointed straight up. Finally, you can stop using an anchor for your feet. This last variation is definitely the hardest of them all, so work your way up to it.

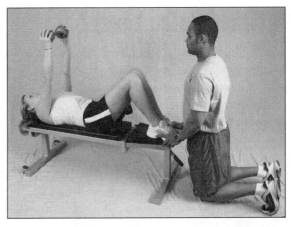

Beginning and ending position on an exercise bench with additional weight held over the head.

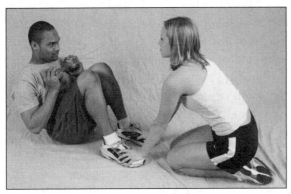

Sit-up with additional weight held against the chest.

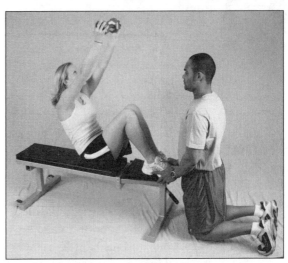

Midpoint of sit-up with weight held over the head.

Inclined Rolls: Level 2

One of my favorite things about gravity is that it is always there to try to push us down. In the case of exercise, this is a good thing. When we push our bodies against gravity, muscles have to work harder than they normally do. Until now, you have done each exercise while lying flat on the floor (at least, your back has been flat). Time to change that. Inclined rolls place your hips higher than your shoulders, so when you perform the movement, you are working uphill.

Spot Me _____

If you have high blood pressure or you get lightheaded easily, these might not be the best exercise for you. Consult your doctor before you try them (basically because more blood gets to your head than you may be used to).

Preparation

1. Grab one or two small throw pillows. Lie on the floor on your back and place the pillows under your hips. Use thin pillows and stack them as feels comfortable. The goal is to get your hips just a little higher than your shoulders. In this case, more isn't necessarily better. Don't use so many pillows that your chin is pressing into your chest—that's bad on your neck.

2. Use your feet to hold the pillows under your butt.

3. Cross your arms over your chest so your fingers rest on your shoulders.

Movement

4. Take a deep breath in. As you exhale, lift your head and roll your shoulders off the ground. You probably won't be able to go as far up as you do with a regular crunch because gravity will push you down off the pillow. Just roll up until you feel yourself start to slide, or until your shoulder blades leave the floor.

5. Breathe in again on the way down, and immediately start another repetition.

Variations

The easiest variation for this exercise is to add more pillows so you work against more gravity.

Level 2: If you are comfortable with the height of your hips, you can hold a small weight against your chest for more resistance.

Level 3: Decrease your base of support by picking up one foot and crossing it over the other one. You've now eliminated half your base of support, while still keeping your back in a good position and making the exercise more challenging.

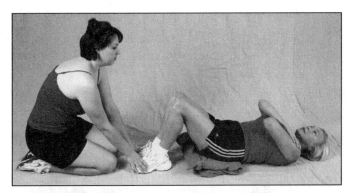

Inclined roll beginning and ending position.

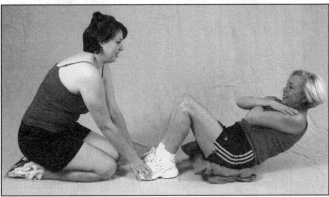

Inclined roll midpoint position.

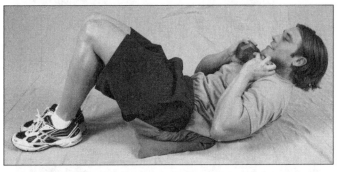

Inclined roll with extra weight on the chest.

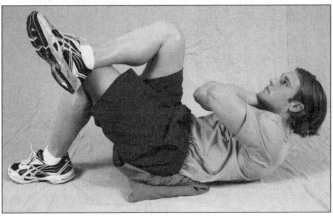

Inclined roll with the legs crossed.

Reverse Crunches: Level 2

Want to approach your abdominal workout from another angle? Try reverse crunches. This exercise works the exact same abdominal muscles as regular crunches, but from a reverse direction. Instead of using the upper-body weight as resistance, the lower body weight fills the role. For each of us, the weight of our upper and lower body differs. For some, the lower body is heavier, while others have more heft higher up. Regardless, this exercise takes advantage of the ability to work the abdominals while teaching you to control your muscles in a different pattern. It takes some work to get the hang of it, but when it happens, you'll definitely know it because you'll feel it.

Preparation

1. Lie on your back on the floor using either an exercise mat or a carpeted surface. Place your hands on the floor next to you, palms down.

2. Tuck your knees up toward your chest.

Movement

3. Take a deep breath in. As you exhale, slowly roll your hips up off the floor, bringing your knees toward your shoulders. Keep your knees as tight against your chest as possible and concentrate on getting the hips just off the floor. This isn't a very big movement, just a slight roll.

In the Mirror _____

No cheating. Don't try to jerk your hips up, don't try to push your feet into the air, and don't push against the floor with your hands.

4. When your hips are off the floor, start breathing in again and slowly lower your hips back down. Immediately start another repetition.

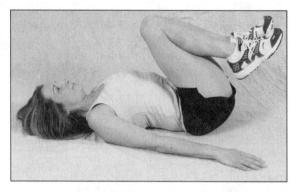

Reverse crunch beginning and ending position.

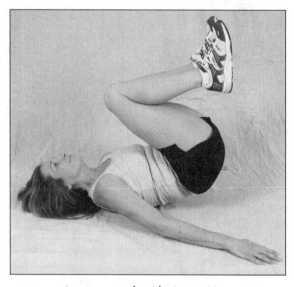

Reverse crunch midpoint position.

Variations

Level 3: Reverse crunches aren't quite enough once you get the hang of it. To entice those abdominal muscles to work even harder for more results, hold your arms out to your sides, just off the floor. This decreases your base of support just enough that you have to work on rolling up and not rolling over at the same time. Talk about a challenge—it's like balancing on your back.

Level 3: If you still feel the need for more, hold your legs straight up in the air with a volleyball or basketball between your feet. Now you have to make sure the legs move together, or else you'll drop the ball.

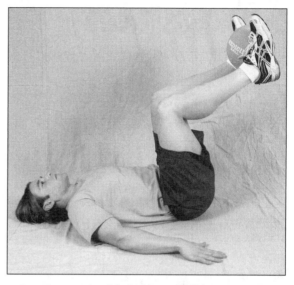

Reverse crunch while holding a ball between your feet, beginning and ending position.

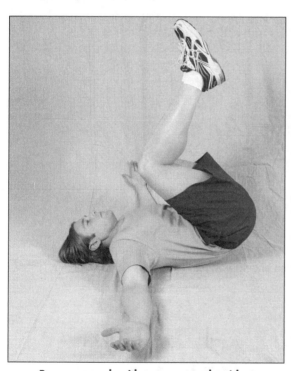

Reverse crunch with arms out to the sides.

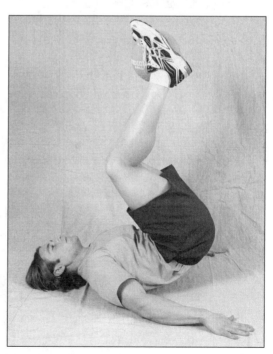

Reverse crunch while holding a ball between your feet, midpoint position.

Double Tucks: Level 3

By now you've tried regular crunches and reverse crunches, so how about putting the two together? That doubles the resistance you have to work with and also makes the abdominal muscles contract about twice as much. It takes a lot of balance and the ability to do two things very well at the same time. If you can handle it—and I'm sure that, with practice, you will—you'll get so much out of this exercise that you'll probably never go back to just one again. (If you haven't gotten the hang of the crunch or reverse crunch, don't try this exercise yet.)

Preparation

1. Lie on your back on an exercise mat or a carpeted surface. Cross your arms over your chest so your fingers touch your shoulders.

2. Lift your knees up and in toward your shoulders. Don't roll your hips up yet, but just relax your lower legs so you aren't holding them up in the air.

Movement

3. Take a deep breath in. As you exhale, perform both a regular crunch and a reverse crunch at the same time. Roll your head and shoulders off the floor, while also rolling your hips off the floor.

4. When you can't crunch up together anymore, breathe in and slowly unroll back to the starting position. Relax for one breath and then begin another repetition.

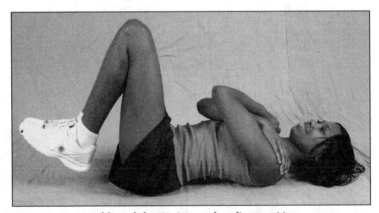

Double tuck beginning and ending position.

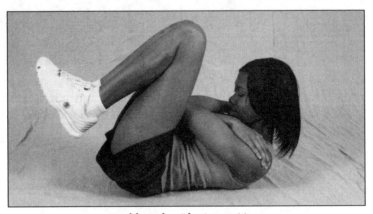

Double tuck midpoint position.

Variations

Level 4: There is only one real way to make this exercise harder: add more resistance. The best way to do that is to hold a small dumbbell or medicine ball in one hand and squeeze

another ball between your feet. Oh, and instead of being tucked, your hands and feet will reach toward the ceiling at the same time while you are crunching.

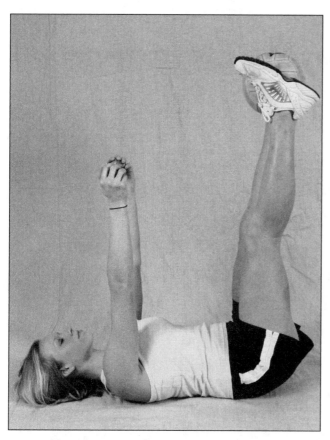

Double tuck variation beginning and ending position.

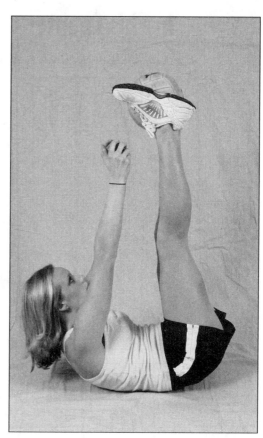

Double tuck variation midpoint position.

In This Chapter

◆ Strengthening and defining your chest

◆ Exercises with just your body weight

◆ Introducing resistance tubing

◆ Isolating one side

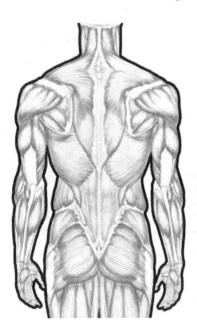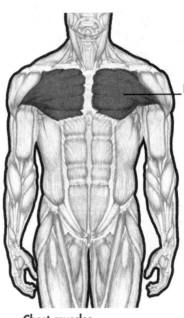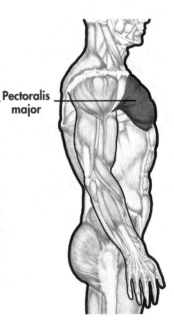

Pectoralis major

Chest muscles.

Chapter 9

Get It Off Your Chest

A knockout workout for your upper body begins with the chest. Although the chest muscle, whose scientific name is the pectoralis major, isn't very visible to the naked eye, the effects it has on the body are completely apparent. This muscle group has the job of controlling your arms during any pushing movement, like opening a door or pushing a grocery cart, and it also defines the shape of your upper chest and part of your shoulders.

One of the largest muscles in the upper body, and one of the strongest, the chest often defines how shirts and suits look on you because these muscles outline the entire area between your shoulders and from your neck to your abdominals. You can show off well-defined pecs (that's what hip people call them) when you wear tank tops, swimsuits, or dresses with plunging necklines. Another neat thing about the chest is that when it moves, the arms move, so you often get several other muscles involved in a little bonus workout. If for no other reason, you should work your pecs because they are the major muscle used when giving hugs.

Wall Press: Level 1

The wall press is the most basic of all the chest exercises and the most specific to real life. Most of the time as we go about our daily activities, we push against things while we are standing up. Examples include opening closed doors, pushing lawnmowers and shopping carts, and pushing through overexcited shoppers during a big sale at Macys. This exercise is basic, but you can make it advanced with some of the variations you'll see, so don't overlook it because it starts off easy.

Preparation

1. Stand close enough to a wall that you can place your hands against it while your arms are totally straight and at shoulder level.

2. Keep your feet together and your body completely rigid—that is, don't let your hips fall forward or your body sag during this exercise.

Movement

3. Bend your arms and slowly lower your chest toward the wall. Stop when your head is about 1 inch from the wall (no leaning your head forward to cheat).

4. Push against the wall with your hands to propel your body back to the starting position.

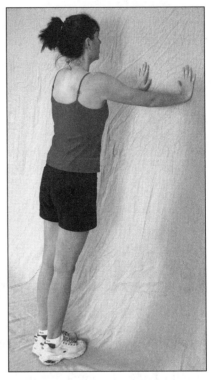

Wall press beginning and ending position.

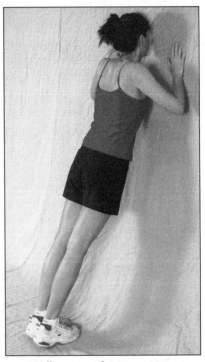

Wall press midpoint position.

Variations

Level 2: Place a small medicine ball against the wall to push against instead of the solid wall. The give of the ball and its ability to move around will make this exercise more challenging.

Level 3: Perform the wall press with only one arm instead of two. Place one hand on the wall right in front of your chest, and hold your other hand behind your back. Now do your repetitions using only one hand. You've doubled the resistance!

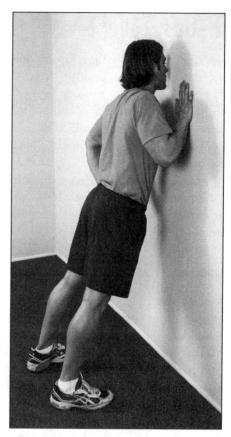

Wall press with only one hand for more resistance.

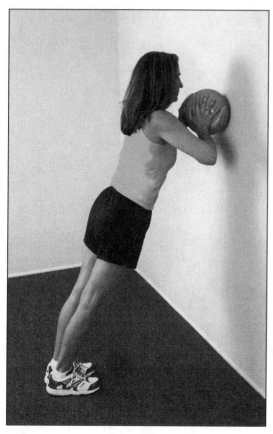

Wall press with a medicine ball for more challenge.

Push-Ups: Level 2

Ranking right up there with sit-ups as one of the oldest exercises is the push-up (maybe all the old exercises have the word *up* in them). Push-ups are cool because they can be done anywhere and without any equipment except for your body. Most people don't like push-ups because they are a little difficult. I say they are only difficult until you start doing them and those chest muscles get stronger. However you look at it, push-ups are a versatile exercise that definitely gets the job done.

Preparation

1. Get down on your hands and knees, and place your hands directly under your shoulders. The wider you put your hands, the harder this exercise becomes and the less your chest actually works, so keep them right at shoulder width. Using fancy push-up handles or doing finger-tip push-ups does nothing to improve this exercise; just a plain old flat hand on the floor is fine.

2. Stretch out your legs and put your feet either right next to each other or no more than a few inches apart. Your toes should be the only part of your body other than your hands to touch the ground, so make sure you have good, solid athletic shoes on.

3. The key to a proper push-up is keeping your body rigid. You want your entire body to move off the ground at one time. Try to maintain a straight line from your shoulders through your hips and to your feet. Don't let your hips sag like an old horse, and don't stick your butt up in the air. Keep your body straight as a board.

Movement

4. Keeping your body straight, slowly bend your arms and lower yourself until either your chest comes in contact with the floor or your shoulders go lower than your elbows. Don't go down so far that you lie on the floor, but get close.

5. Push against your hands to lift your body back up to the point that your arms are straight again.

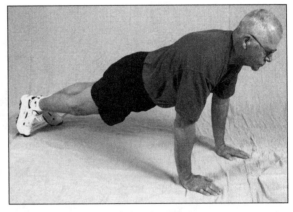

Push-up beginning and ending position.

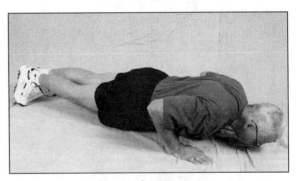

Push-up midpoint position.

Variations

Level 1: If you have trouble doing enough repetitions of the basic push-up, try the modified version until you build up some more chest strength. Instead of pivoting from your toes, put your knees on the ground and bend your knees. This allows you to lift only the weight of your body from your knees to your head, and it changes the physics of the exercise to allow you to get stronger before moving on.

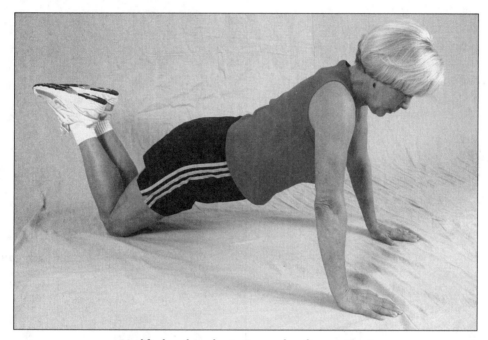

Modified push-up beginning and ending position.

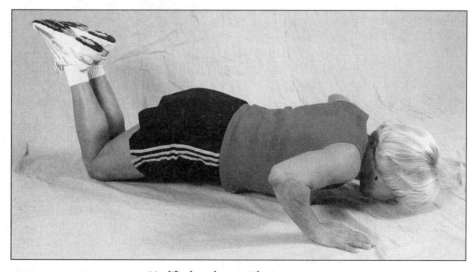

Modified push-up midpoint position.

Tubing Press: Level 1

The tubing press is a great way to work your chest if you don't have any heavy equipment and can't get down on the floor for push-ups. Tubing presses are a little different than the other chest exercises because the farther you stretch resistance tubing, the harder the exercise becomes. This is ideal for working the chest because you can actually handle more weight as your hands move farther away from you. Anytime you use tubing, you have a versatile way of increasing resistance: just shorten the tubing for a harder workout.

Preparation

1. Anchor the tubing by wrapping it around a pole or a doorknob, or something heavy that won't come flying at you when you pull on it.

2. Hold one end of the tubing in each hand, and face away from your anchor. Lift your elbows and hold your hands just under your shoulders.

3. Put one foot in front of the other to create a solid base. As you push out on the tubing, it will try to pull you back. Positioning your feet solidly on the ground will keep you from moving.

Movement

4. Press out with both hands until your arms are straight.

5. Slowly bend your elbows and bring your hands back to their starting position near your shoulders. The tubing will try to pull you back quickly, so control the return to the starting position without being yanked back.

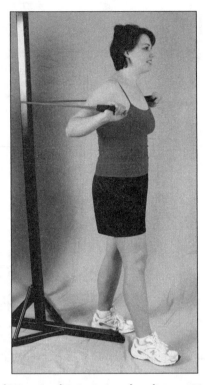

Tubing press beginning and ending position.

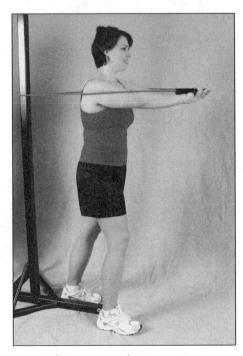

Tubing press midpoint position.

Variations

Level 1: Instead of moving both arms at the same time, you can alternate left and right side repetitions. Hold the tubing in place just like normal, but keep one hand at the shoulder while the other hand presses out.

Level 2: To increase the resistance, you can put both handles in one hand and do a set of single arm presses with twice the resistance. Place your other hand on your hip to keep it out of the way.

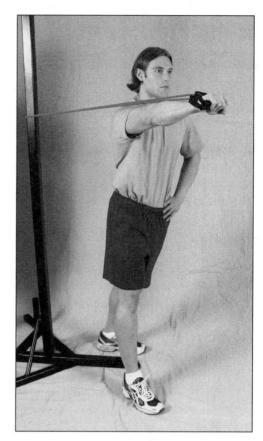

Double the resistance with both handles in one hand.

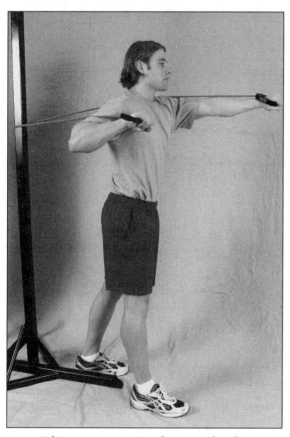

Tubing press variation alternating hands.

Machine Press: Level 1

Machines are excellent choices for working the chest muscles because they control the direction of the movement so you don't have to fiddle with balance and coordination. Depending on what brand of equipment you are using, the chest press machine goes by many names: vertical chest press, seated chest press, seated bench press, and, as one of my clients likes to call it, "That hard one where you push out."

Preparation

1. Proper seat adjustment is the key to maximizing the effects of the chest press. Sitting too low or too high won't feel right and looks just plain funny. Imagine that there is a solid bar running across your chest from each of the handles. You want this bar to be at chest height, not neck height or stomach height. Adjust the seat up or down to achieve this position.

2. Most of the newer chest-press machines have two sets of handles, a horizontal set and a vertical set. Ignore the vertical set; this is used for another exercise. Grab the horizontal handles and lift your elbows so they are the same height as your hands and shoulders. If you let your elbows hang down, you force your shoulder muscles to do most of the work. You want to focus on the chest, so lift those elbows high.

3. Sit up straight in the chair—no slouching. Keep your back flat against the pad and your feet flat on the ground.

Movement

4. Push the handles out until your arms are completely straight.

5. Slowly bend your elbows and let the handles come back toward your shoulders until the weights almost touch the stack, but not quite. You don't want the weights to come to a rest. Keeping the weight up in the air a bit keeps the muscles working longer. Now just push it back out for another rep.

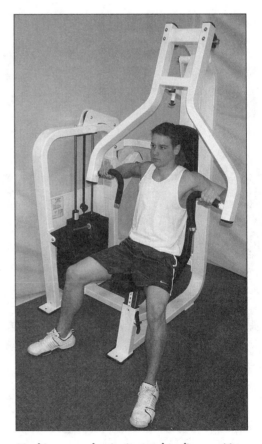

Machine press beginning and ending position.

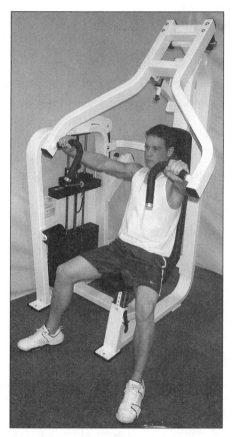

Machine press midpoint position.

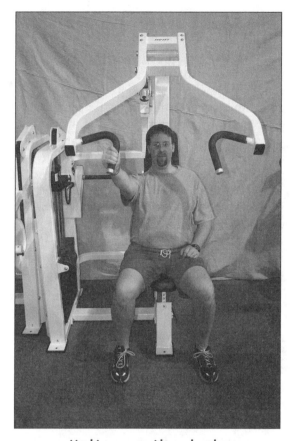

Machine press with one hand.

Variations

Level 2: You can use machines to work one side of your chest at a time. Keep one hand in your lap and go through the motions with the other hand; then switch so you don't get lopsided results. The benefit of working one side at a time is that you can focus on improving your weak side by doing a few more reps than your strong side.

Dumbbell Press: Level 2

The dumbbell press is an excellent exercise that allows you to work on your strength in combination with your balance and coordination. Lifting two weights in the air can get a bit tricky, so start with relatively light weight and get comfortable with the movement before tackling any heavy lifting. One of the key elements in the dumbbell press is balancing the weights so they move up and down together smoothly. Since we all have a dominant side that is a little stronger, you may feel that one side of your body is not working as hard, but that's okay. With time, the dumbbell press will train your weaker side to catch up, and you won't be lopsided anymore.

Spot Me

Since you will be holding weights in the air over your head, it's important to have a spotter to assist you.

Preparation

1. Lie on your back on an exercise bench or aerobics step with a dumbbell in each hand. Keep both feet on the floor, and keep your hips, butt, and shoulders on the bench.
2. Start the exercise by placing the dumbbells in a resting position on each shoulder, with your elbows out to the side.

Movement

3. Press the dumbbells straight up in the air over your chest until your arms are completely straight. Don't allow the dumbbells to hover over your head or down by your stomach—they should always be directly over your chest and shoulders.
4. Slowly lower the dumbbells back down to your shoulders.
5. While the dumbbells are moving up and down, they should follow a straight, smooth path. If you see them moving out to the sides in a circular path to the top, bring them back in line. Moving the dumbbells out to the sides forces your biceps to work too much and uses extra energy.

Variations

Level 1: Instead of lying on a bench, lie on the floor. This decreases the range of motion and concentrates your efforts on the last half of the motion, where it is usually the hardest. Start with your elbows resting on the floor, dumbbells directly over the elbows. Push up to a point directly over your chest and return to the floor.

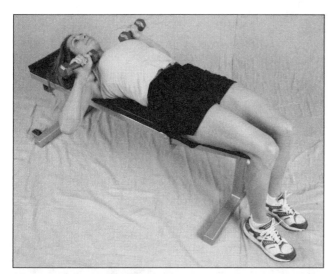

Dumbbell press beginning and ending position.

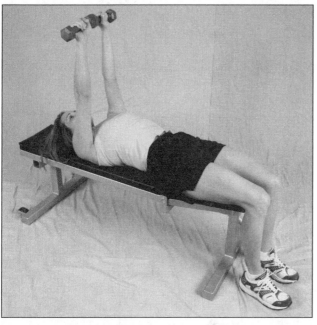

Dumbbell press midpoint position.

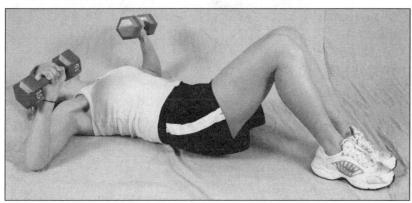

Beginning and ending position
for dumbbell press on the floor.

Bench Press: Level 3

The renowned bench press is the granddaddy of all chest exercises. As one of the first organized exercises that men competed in, the bench press continues to elicit a great deal of awe and envy to this day—particularly as the weights get higher. Magazines place a lot of emphasis on the bench press, but each of the exercises in this chapter works the same muscles, so the bench press doesn't have to be a part of your knockout workout. It's a good exercise, but it isn't a "better than anything else" exercise.

Preparation

1. Lie down on the bench (on your back), and keep your feet on the floor.
2. Place your hands on the bar approximately shoulder width apart. The small marking rings around the bar are to help you make sure your hands are an equal distance from the middle of the bar, so use them as reference points.

Spot Me

Since the bar will be over your head and chest, make sure you have a spotter to assist you.

Movement

3. Lift the bar off its resting hooks and hold it over your chest. Don't let it move over your head or down over your stomach. At a certain point, your arms will be perfectly vertical and the bar will feel relatively light.
4. Slowly lower the bar to about an inch above your chest. Keep the bar away from your head and neck.

5. Push the bar back up until your arms are straight again. As you push, move the bar in a straight line. If you feel the bar moving more toward your head or stomach, make adjustments to keep it positioned over your chest.

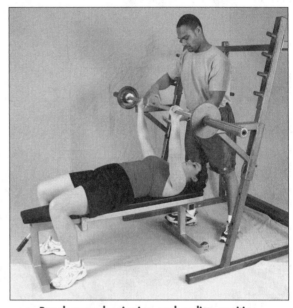

Bench press beginning and ending position.

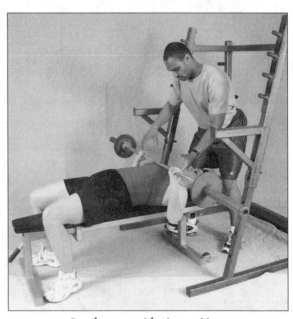

Bench press midpoint position.

Variations

Level 4: You can increase the range of motion your chest works through and increase the difficulty of the exercise by using a grip that is narrower than shoulder width. Place your hands about 6 inches apart in the middle of the bar. This increases the balance and coordination efforts of this exercise, and decreases the weight you can use.

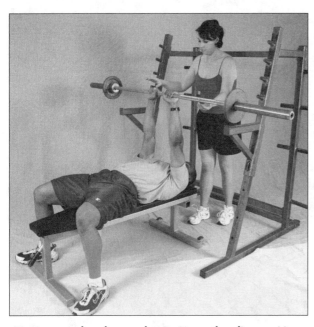

Narrow grip bench press beginning and ending position.

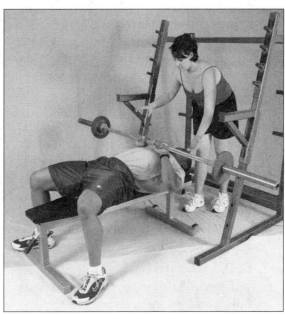

Narrow grip bench press midpoint position.

Incline Press: Level 2

The incline press changes the emphasis of the exercise from just the chest muscles and increases your use of the front portion of the shoulder muscles. It's still a chest exercise, but you get some help from the shoulders, which adds to the results of the exercise and gives a larger part of your chest and shoulders a knockout look.

Preparation

1. Lie on an inclined exercise bench. The incline of most benches is about 45°, but this can vary a little without any real difference in results. You can use either an adjustable bench or a special fixed-incline bench; it really doesn't matter as long as your head is higher than your hips in the starting position.

2. Grab hold of the bar with a shoulder-width grip. Lift the bar off the rack and hold it straight up in the air over your chest.

Spot Me _____

With a bar over your head and chest, you'll need a spotter for this exercise.

Movement

3. Slowly lower the bar to within an inch of your chest. As you lower the bar, don't let it come down over your head or stomach—keep it over your chest.

4. Push the bar back up to the starting position, keeping it smooth and steady.

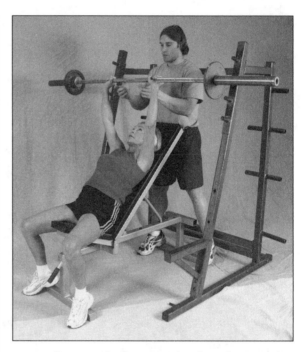

Incline press beginning and ending position.

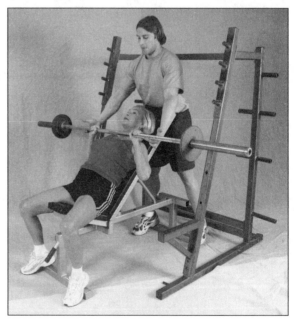

Incline press midpoint position.

Variations

Level 2: The incline press can also be done with dumbbells. Hold a dumbbell in each hand at your shoulders, press the dumbbells straight up until the arms are fully extended, and then slowly let them back down. Remember to push with each arm evenly.

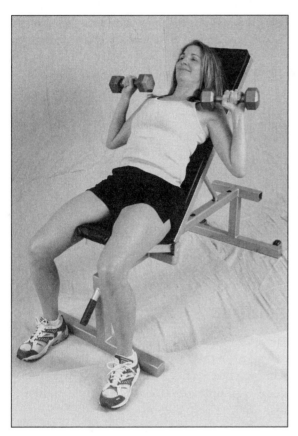

Incline press with dumbbells beginning and ending position.

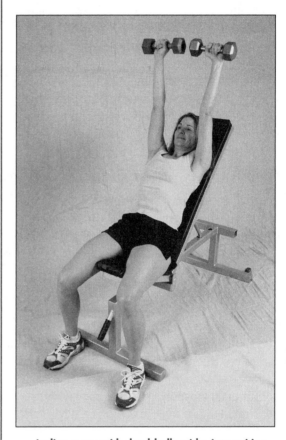

Incline press with dumbbells midpoint position.

Machine Fly: Level 1

The machine fly is a great exercise to watch in the mirror. I tell clients to pretend they are flexing their muscles like the bodybuilders on TV do. The fly exercise isolates the chest muscles like no other exercise does. The shoulders and arms can't help, so the chest has to work harder than usual; this means you can use a lighter weight than with a pressing exercise. This exercise really shows off the muscles in your chest and shoulders that you've been working so hard for, so enjoy the results.

Preparation

1. Adjust the seat to its proper height. As in the machine press, pretend there is a solid bar from one handle to the other. This bar should pass right across your chest. Adjust the seat up or down to achieve this position.

2. Depending on the brand of machine, you may also be able to adjust how far back the handles go. If they're back too far, you risk injury. But if they're not back far enough, you may miss out on part of the exercise. Adjust the handles so that your hands are stretched out to your sides, but never farther back than your shoulders (any farther back puts your shoulder stability at risk).

3. Keep your arms straight, with just a slight bend in the elbows. This is not a pressing exercise, but a fly, so think big, long wings. Sit up straight and keep your feet on the floor.

Movement

4. Pretend that you are hugging a giant tree. Maintain a slight bend in your elbows and bring your arms out and together. This exercise is called a fly for a reason: think about flapping your arms like a bird. Slowly bring your hands together far out in front of you.

5. When your hands meet, slowly return the weight to the starting position. Be sure not to let the weight completely rest on the weight stack before your next rep.

 In the Mirror

You may feel a need to lean forward during this exercise if you get tired. Don't. Keep your back flat against the pad and keep your head out of the way of the arms of the machine.

Variations

Level 2: You can work one side of your chest at a time on this machine. Simply place one hand in your lap while the other arm works. To get even more out of this single-arm variation, instead of stopping when your arm is straight out in front of you, bring it as far across your body as you can.

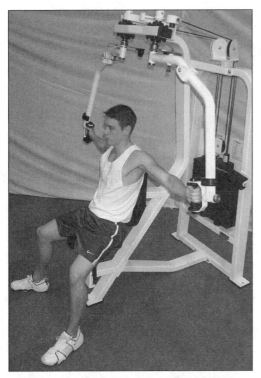

Machine fly beginning and ending position.

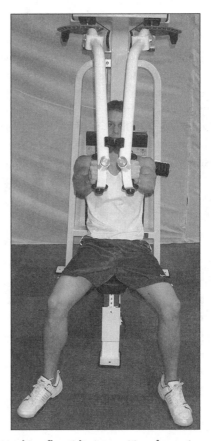

Machine fly midpoint position, front view.

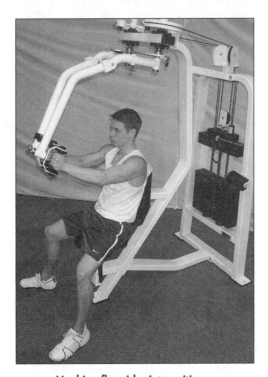

Machine fly midpoint position.

Dumbbell Fly: Level 3

The dumbbell fly is a lot like the machine fly, in that it isolates the chest muscles. However, it is an advanced exercise because you really have to control the weight during the descent, and coordinate the movements of both your arms while balancing on the bench. This is a great exercise for really getting deep into the chest muscles and making every single fiber work to its max.

Preparation

1. Lie on an exercise bench. Place your feet on top of the bench. This requires some balance, so make sure you feel comfortable in this position.
2. Hold a pair of dumbbells straight up over your chest.

Spot Me

Be sure to have a spotter any time you have dumbbells over your head or chest.

Movement

3. Keep a slight bend in your elbows as you let the dumbbells move apart and toward the floor in a big arc. Don't bend the elbows any more as the weight goes down. Try to keep the dumbbells as far away from you as possible at all times. Lower the dumbbells until they are level with your shoulders.

4. Use those chest muscles to pull the dumbbells back to their starting position above your chest. This movement should resemble an arc, not a straight-line press. Make sure they move at the same speed so one side isn't finished before the other.

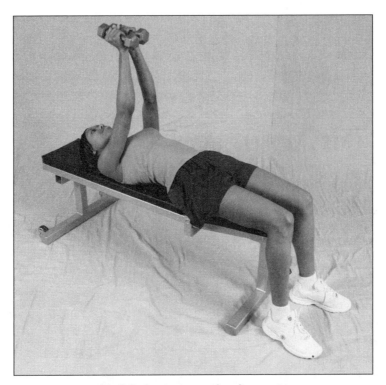

Dumbbell fly beginning and ending position.

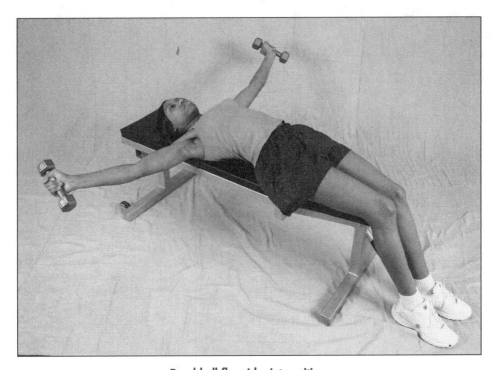

Dumbbell fly midpoint position.

In This Chapter

- ◆ Pulling with your back
- ◆ Creating that tapered look
- ◆ Isolate for more results
- ◆ Learning to do chin-ups

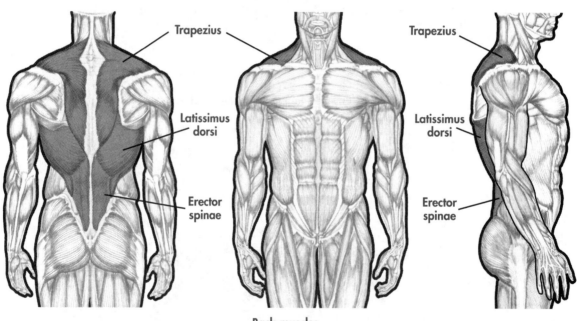

Back muscles.

Chapter 10

Coming Back for More

You may not have ever thought so, but your back can be one of the most knockout parts of your whole body. Don't believe me? Think about the last time you saw someone in a strapless or spaghetti-strap dress or swimsuit, or your own bare back in the mirror. Could you see the individual muscles or just a smooth layer of fat covering them? When they moved, were the shoulder blades sticking out strangely? A knockout back doesn't have to be about well-defined muscles, but it probably isn't about having little rolls of fat under your armpits and shoulder blades, either.

The knockout exercises in this chapter are designed to do two things: 1) make your back look great, and 2) make your back strong. A knockout workout incorporates exercises that highlight the natural shape of your back, which is a taper from your shoulders to your waist. The back has a lot of muscles (see the picture to the left), so there's a lot of work to do.

Even worse than not liking the way your back looks is dealing with constant annoying back pain (yes, I have hurt my back before, and it's no fun). It's estimated that more than half the American population has back pain. Good thing back pain is often linked to weak muscles—we can fix that and make your back look incredible at the same time.

Pull-Ups and Chin-Ups: Level 1

Most people don't know that there is a difference between a pull-up and a chin-up. Both exercises use basically the same muscles, but the hand position is different. I know, that's not a big difference, but it does change the exercise a little. With chin-ups, you use a bit more of your biceps muscles than in a pull-up—just a little, but it may make the difference of a couple extra repetitions. You'll also notice that I labeled this exercise as a Level 1. I did this knowing that most people cannot do even one chin-up or pull-up. So why Level 1? Because the exercise technique is simple, and everyone can improve and get better at it with hard work.

Preparation

1. Find a pull-up/chin-up bar that's at least a couple of inches higher than you can reach. If you can reach the bar without jumping up to get it, be sure to bend your knees while doing this exercise—otherwise, you will touch the ground at the bottom of each repetition.

2. For a pull-up, grab hold of the bar with a grip that's slightly wider than shoulder width, palms facing away from you. For a chin-up, grab the bar so your hands are about 6 inches apart, palms facing toward you. Look at the pictures for clarification.

3. Hang from the bar and let your back completely stretch out.

Movement

4. Pull yourself up to the bar. Try to get your chin all the way to the bar (and no cheating by lifting your chin and stretching your neck). If you can't get all the way up right now, that's fine; just go as far as you can. I promise you'll get there if you keep working at it.

5. When you get to the top, don't stop and admire the view. Slowly lower yourself back down and get ready for the next rep.

Spot Me _____

During this exercise, be sure to lower your body slowly. Dropping quickly can overextend your elbows, which can be very painful.

Variations

Level 1: If you are having problems getting all the way up to the bar, you can reverse this exercise and start at the top. Use a stool to help you up into the midpoint position, and then slowly lower yourself to the ground. Working the muscles in reverse will make them stronger and will help you get to the point that you can do a regular pull-up or chin-up.

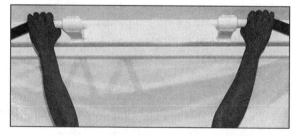

Pull-up hand position.

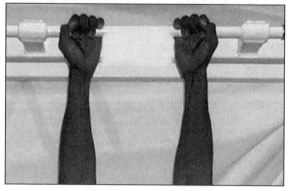

Chin-up hand position.

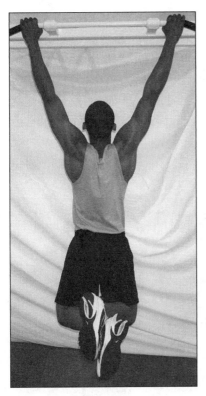

Pull-up beginning and ending position.

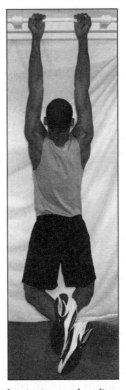

Chin-up beginning and ending position.

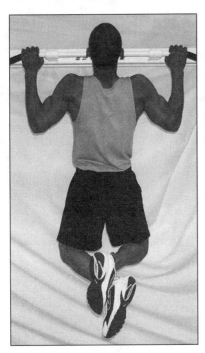

Pull-up midpoint position.

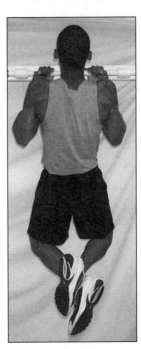

Chin-up midpoint position.

Lying Pull-Ups: Level 1

The lying pull-up is a interesting exercise that's part of the President's Physical Fitness Test that kids take in school, more trainers are starting to use it with their adult clients. It's really neat because it uses your body weight against gravity for the resistance, and it trains the same muscles you use to pull open doors, drag the garbage out to the street, and make the top part of your back extremely sexy.

Preparation

1. This exercise requires a bar just high enough to reach while lying on the ground. I usually use a squat bar resting on the low hooks of a squat cage. Look around where you work out to find something similar.

2. Lie on the floor under the bar and use either a pull-up or chin-up grip. Adjust yourself on the floor so that your arms are slightly angled toward your feet (about 20° or so).

3. Place your feet together, with the rest of your body lying stretched out. Think of this as the opposite of a push-up. At rest, you are essentially in the same position as the start/finish position of the push-up (except on your back).

Movement

4. Pull yourself up until your chest reaches the bar. As you pull, your entire body should leave the ground at one time. It may help to pretend you are lying on a board that makes a straight line from your shoulders, through your hips, and down to your feet.

5. Slowly lower yourself back to the floor. You can actually rest on the floor between reps, if you like (just try not to take a nap).

Spot Me

To avoid falling from the bar, stop if you feel weak or if sweat is causing your hands to slip.

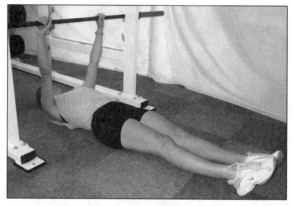

Lying pull-up beginning and ending position.

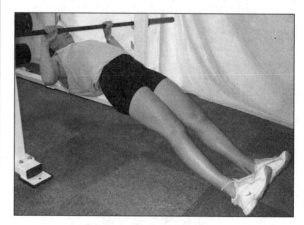

Lying pull-up midpoint position.

Variations

Level 1: If you don't have a bar you can use, attach your resistance tubing to something above you (like the top of a door) and use that for the resistance. Instead of pulling yourself up off the floor, you'll pull the tubing down to you. Just make sure you adjust the resistance of the tubing to make this exercise difficult enough.

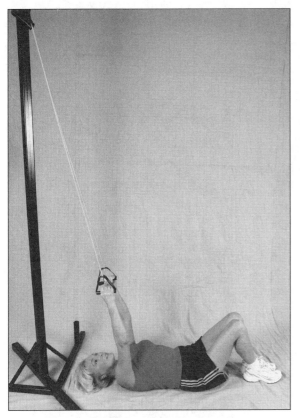

Lying pull-up with resistance tubing beginning and ending position.

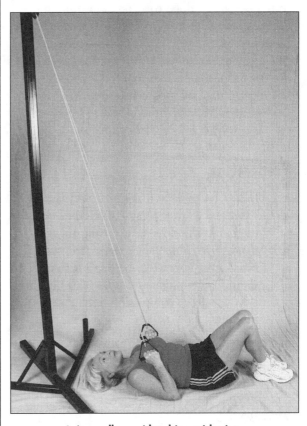

Lying pull-up with tubing midpoint.

Lat Pulldowns: Level 1

The lat pulldown has to be the most popular back machine in the gym (remember that popular doesn't make it the best). This exercise works the largest muscle in your back, known as the latissimus dorsi (or lats). This muscle reaches across most of your middle back and allows you to move your arms close to your body. Any time you pull on something, the lats are the hardest-working muscles. This is also the muscle that gives your back a tapered look because it is wider at the top and narrows as it travels down to your erector spinae muscles.

Preparation

1. Find a lat-pulldown machine with a long bar attached to the cable. Grab hold of the bar at shoulder width using an overhand grip (palms facing away from you). No matter how wide the bar is, use only a shoulder-width grip—any wider will prevent you from completing a full range of motion.

2. Sit in the seat and place your knees under the pad. The pad gives you some leverage to help pull the bar down.

Movement

3. Starting with your arms completely straight, pull the bar down in front of your face until it reaches your chin.

4. Slowly let the bar back up, making sure your arms are fully extended before the next repetition.

Spot Me

Never pull the bar down behind your head. This is a common mistake in this exercise that usually results in a shoulder injury.

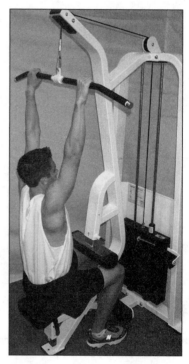

Lat pulldown beginning and ending position.

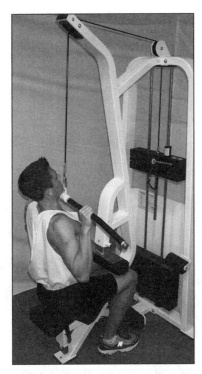

Lat pulldown midpoint position.

Variations

Level 1: Switch to an underhand grip (palms facing you). Although the movement is the same, this grip will allow you to also work your biceps, and you may be able to handle more weight.

Level 1: You can also use a narrow v-grip bar. If you have wrist problems, the v-grip bar is easier because it places your hands in a neutral position (palms facing each other).

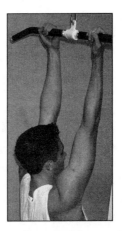

Lat pulldown performed with an underhand grip.

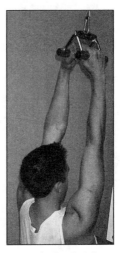

Lat pulldown performed with a v-grip bar.

Seated Row: Level 2

This exercise is the first you will perform with a cable/pulley machine. The seated row works a combination of the big lat muscles and the smaller erector spinae muscles lower in the back. The spinae muscles are responsible for your posture and lower-back strength. When you slouch in your chair, it's because either those muscles aren't doing their job well enough or you're just a little lazy (just kidding, but made you sit up, didn't I?).

Preparation

1. Find the low-pulley machine at your gym. If you don't have one, turn to the tubing row a little later in this chapter for a variation that you can do without a machine. Sit down on the bench and grab hold of the v-grip handle that should be attached to the cable.

2. Put your feet against the platforms at the base of the machine, and scoot back until your legs are almost straight.

3. Holding on to the handle, sit as straight as you can.

Movement

4. Keep your back straight while you pull the handle all the way to your stomach. Concentrate on keeping your elbows close to your sides as you pull back.

5. Slowly let the handle back out, but don't let your body lean forward—keep that straight posture.

Spot Me

If you experience any pulling or pain in your lower back during this exercise, stop and consult your doctor before you try it again.

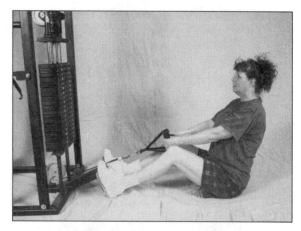

Seated row beginning and ending position.

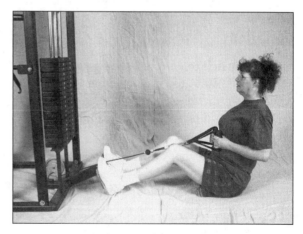

Seated row midpoint position.

Variations

Level 1: Use your resistance tubing instead of a cable/pulley machine. Attach your tubing to a pole about a foot off the ground. Hold one handle in each hand, sit on the floor, and scoot back until there is some stretch in the tubing before you start. Sit straight and pull the handles to your stomach. Slowly let them out again and repeat. Remember to stay sitting straight the entire time.

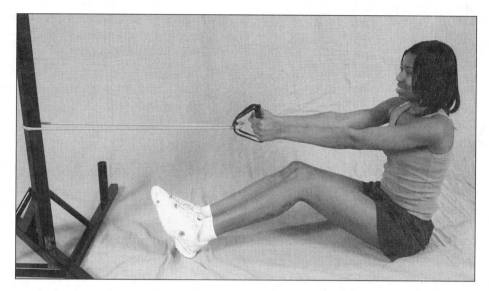

Seated row with resistance tubing beginning and ending position.

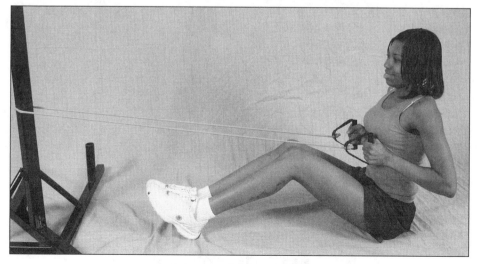

Seated row with tubing midpoint.

Tubing Row: Level 2

Okay, you've done a bunch of seated back exercises, so it's time you stood up for a while. When you pull with the back muscles while you are standing, you have to work a little differently to keep from falling forward. Your legs brace you while your upper back does all the work. In between your legs and your upper back are those posture muscles called the erector spinae. They are at it again, trying to keep your back nice and straight while you pull on stuff. That's their job, and if you keep training this way, they are likely to get really good at it and make you look even better—after all, you never see a knockout body that slouches.

Preparation

1. Attach your tubing to a pole, door, or heavy machine about chest high.

2. Hold one handle in each hand and step back while holding your arms out in front of you. Keep moving back until there is a little stretch in the tubing to start. Stand with one foot in front of the other for a good base of support.

Movement

3. Hold your elbows at shoulder level as you pull back on both handles. Pull back as far as you can, hopefully until your hands reach your shoulders. Keep those elbows up and out to the sides.

4. Slowly let the tubing back out without letting it pull you forward. Keep your back straight and still.

Variations

Level 1: To reduce the effect of the tubing trying to pull you forward, keep your elbows at your sides as you pull your hands back to your stomach. This looks a lot like the seated row, except that you have to stand straight the whole time.

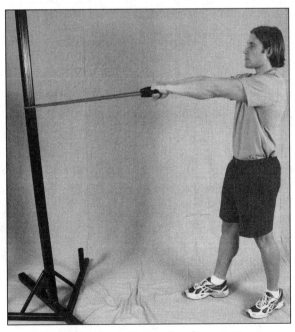

Tubing row beginning and ending position.

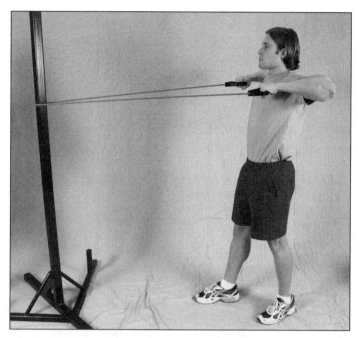

Tubing row midpoint position.

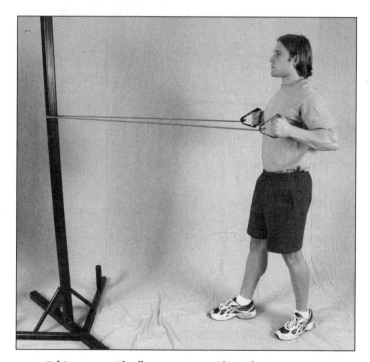

Tubing row with elbows at your side midpoint position.

Bent-Over Row: Level 3

The bent-over row is one of the most challenging exercises for the lower back—especially since the lower back isn't even moving during this exercise. Any time you lean forward, the erector spinae muscles have to double or triple the work they do to keep your back straight—that's a lot of effort from some little muscles. So how's this make you look any better? Easy—the lower-back muscles are allowing the upper back to become more sculpted by supporting them during their work.

Spot Me

The bent-over row is an advanced exercise that can be trouble for anyone with back problems. If your back isn't 100 percent, skip this exercise for now.

Preparation

1. Hold a dumbbell in each hand. Stand with one foot slightly in front of the other. Bend forward at the waist. Keep your back as straight as possible.

2. Keep leaning forward until your upper body is at about a 45° angle, or until you cannot keep your back straight anymore. Let your arms hang straight down.

Movement

3. Keep your elbows close to your body as you pull the dumbbells up to your stomach.

4. Slowly let your arms straighten out again.

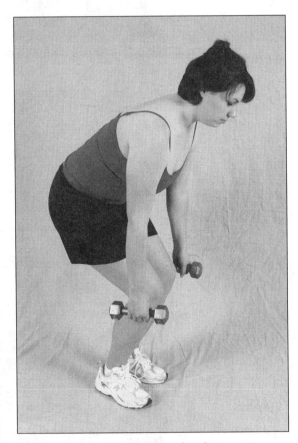

Bent-over row beginning and ending position.

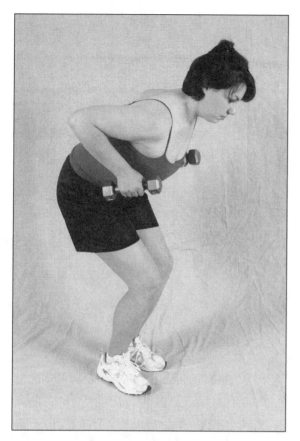

Bent-over row midpoint.

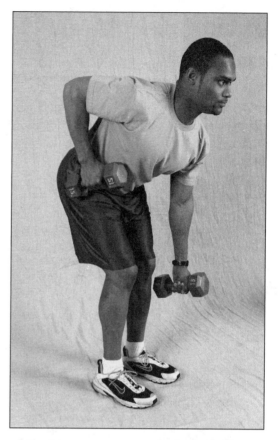

Bent-over row one arm at a time midpoint.

Variations

Level 3: You can work one side of your upper back at a time by completing a full set with one arm and then a full set with the other. When one arm is working, the other arm is hanging straight, waiting its turn.

Straight-Arm Pulldown: Level 2

Few exercises can isolate the big lat muscles in the back without involving the biceps during the movement. The straight-arm pulldown does just that. Here is your chance to see exactly what your back muscles are capable of, force them to really work, and, as a result, make them look amazing. You won't need a lot of weight for this exercise—actually, less than you've used so far. Without the biceps to assist, the focus is on just one muscle, so isolate and appreciate.

Preparation

1. Stand facing a high-pulley machine with either a straight bar or a pair of single handles attached up high. If you don't have this machine, you can attach your resistance tubing to the top of a door and achieve the same result.

2. Step back so that your hands start above your head, arms straight. Place one foot in front of the other to provide a solid base of support.

Movement

3. Push down against your hands so that the bar travels down and toward your thighs. Keep you arms straight the whole time so your body can pivot at the shoulders.

4. Stop when your hands reach your thighs, and slowly let the bar/handles back up to the starting position.

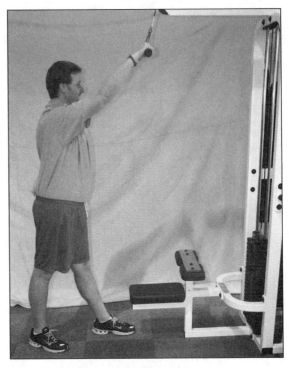

Straight arm pulldown beginning and ending position.

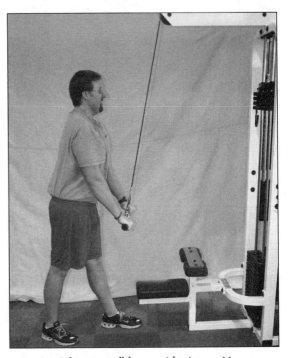

Straight arm pulldown midpoint position.

Variations

Level 1: You can work one side of your back at a time by using only a single handle and moving only one arm. The other hand should rest against your hip to keep it out of the way. Remember to lighten the load by about half.

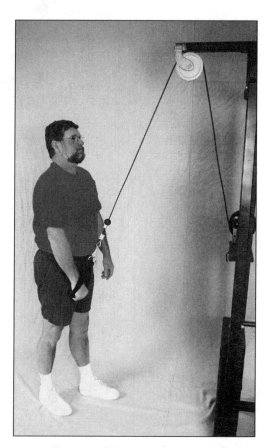

Straight arm pulldown using only one arm.

Pullovers: Level 3

Finally, you can make the straight arm pulldown exercise that isolates the back muscles even better by taking the rest of your body out of the equation. The pullover is done lying down so your legs, abdominals, and lower back don't have to work to keep your posture correct. This is the most isolating exercise I can think of for the upper back, and it can surely bring that knockout look to everyone.

Preparation

1. Lie on your back on an exercise bench. Hold a single dumbbell with both hands directly over your chest, arms straight.

2. Place your feet on the bench to keep your back as straight as possible. If you don't feel comfortable with your feet on the bench (if you feel like you might roll off), do this exercise lying on an aerobic bench with your feet on the floor.

Movement

3. Slowly lower the dumbbell out over the bench behind your head. Lower it only to about the same level of your head, or to the point that you feel your back start to really arch.

4. Using the muscles in your back, pull the dumbbell back to the starting position. Remember to keep your arms straight all the time.

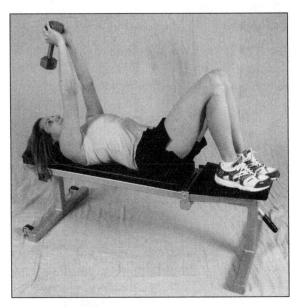

Pullover beginning and ending position.

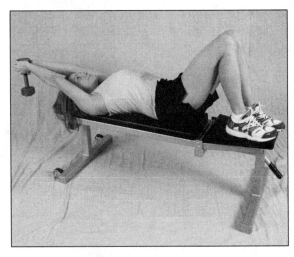

Pullover midpoint position.

Spot Me _____

This is another exercise for which having a spotter is a good idea. Even a single dumbbell can hurt and possibly cause injury if you drop it on your head or chest.

Variations

Level 3: You may choose to use a barbell instead of a dumbbell for the resistance. Hold a barbell with your hands about shoulder width apart. Make sure you use a closed grip (thumb wrapped around the barbell opposite of the fingers) so the bar can't slip out of your hands.

Level 2: You can also do this exercise with resistance tubing. Attach one end of the tubing to the bottom of a door or pole. Hold the other handle in both hands. Since the tubing will have the most stretch when it is over your chest, begin this version with your hands already over your head, and pull it up over your chest (exactly the opposite of the dumbbell and barbell versions).

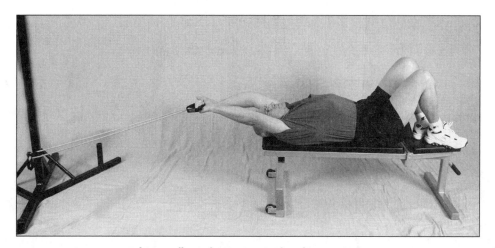

Tubing pullover beginning and ending position.

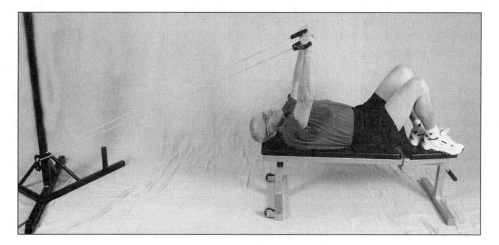

Tubing pullover midpoint position.

In This Chapter

◆ The three parts of the shoulder

◆ Emphasizing and isolating

◆ The muscle you can't see, but *they* can

◆ A military exercise

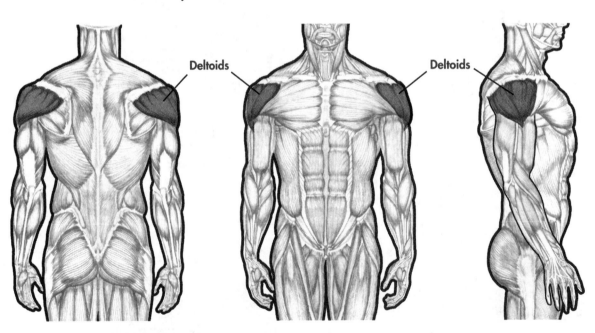

Shoulder muscles.

11

The World on Your Shoulders

Your shoulders are often one of the most noticed parts of your upper body. If you don't believe me, explain why someone invented shoulder pads for suits and blouses. Knockout shoulders are almost expected, so get rid of those pads and make your muscles stand up and be recognized.

Every movement your arms make requires the shoulder to move as well, so a strong and well-defined shoulder will help make your entire upper body look even better. You can't do any chest or back exercise without also working the shoulder, so they get a little bit of a workout with other exercises. But we isolate them as much as possible in this chapter.

If you look at the picture of the deltoid muscle on the opposite page, you'll notice that it has small lines running through it. This muscle actually has three distinct parts that can be emphasized to different extents with each exercise. The front portion of your deltoid is usually the strongest, since most of the movements you do in normal life are in front of you. The side, or middle, portion of the deltoid is responsible for lifting your arm out to the side, and it is also quite strong. The back portion of the deltoid does a lot of work during the back exercises, but it is still part of the shoulder, so we'll be sure to give it a good workout, too.

Front Raise: Level 1

I think dumbbells are the best tool to use for your shoulders because they allow your arms to move independently of each other. Some trainers suggest doing this exercise with both arms at the same time, but I believe it's more effective to concentrate and isolate one shoulder at a time. This exercise isolates the front portion of your deltoid the most, which is the part you primarily use for everyday tasks such as picking things up and reaching out. Do this exercise in front of a mirror to see the definition with each repetition.

Preparation

1. Stand with your feet slightly apart, one foot in front of the other.
2. Hold a dumbbell in each hand, with your palms facing your legs.

Movement

3. Start with either arm, and slowly lift the dumbbell straight out in front of you until it's at eye level. Keep your arm as straight as possible.
4. Slowly lower the dumbbell back to your leg and repeat with the other arm, alternating back and forth until you have finished your set.

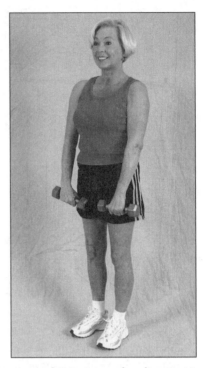

Front raise beginning and ending position.

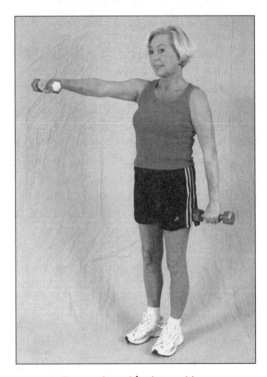

Front raise midpoint position.

Variations

Level 1: You can also use resistance tubing for this exercise. Stand on the middle of the tubing to anchor it, and hold one handle in each hand. Now lift one arm at a time to eye level and back down. With tubing, the resistance increases the higher you lift it. If you can't get your arm up all the way because the tubing is too tight, adjust the tubing so there is less tension on it at the beginning of the exercise, and complete a set with one arm at a time instead of alternating left and right.

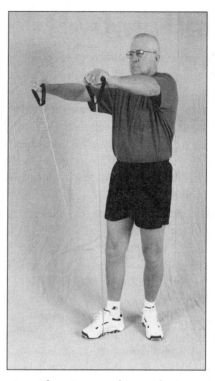

Front raise with resistance tubing midpoint position.

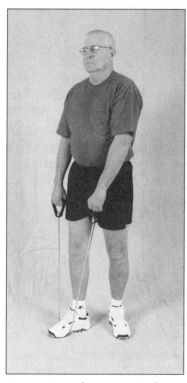

Front raise with resistance tubing beginning and ending position.

Lateral Raise: Level 1

The lateral raise emphasizes the middle or side part of the deltoid muscle a bit more. Not very many of the motions we do in everyday life involve lifting something to the side of the body, so why is this exercise worth your time? The side portion of the deltoid provides some support for both the front and rear portions of the same muscle. If you leave it weak, it can't do its job. On top of that, to have a well-rounded looking shoulder, you have to work every part of it; you can't forget even the smallest, least-used side. Oh, and did I mention how great this muscle looks when you do work it out? And that's the whole point anyway, right?

Preparation

1. Stand with your feet apart, one foot slightly behind the other for balance.

2. Hold a dumbbell in each hand against the outside of your thighs, palms facing your legs.

Movement

3. Keep your arms straight or just slightly bent at the elbow. Lift both arms out to your sides until the dumbbells are shoulder height. You have to do this exercise with both arms at the same time, to prevent unnecessary strain on your back.

4. Slowly lower your arms back to your sides. Though you may be tempted to simply let your arms drop, you'll lose half the effectiveness of the exercise by neglecting to work your muscles on the way down, too.

Spot Me

If you feel any shoulder pain, or if you have been diagnosed with shoulder impingement, lift the dumbbell only as high as you can without experiencing pain. Don't "work through" the pain; this may only lead to additional injury.

Variations

Level 1: Of course, you can do this exercise with resistance tubing as well. Stand on the middle of the tubing to anchor it. Hold one handle in each hand and lift both arms to shoulder height. Since you will be stretching the tubing in both directions, the resistance may jump up pretty high. You may have to use a lighter resistance tube for this exercise.

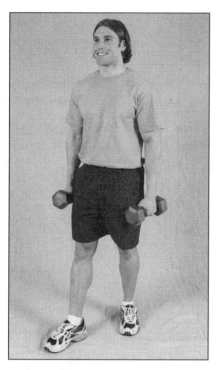

Lateral raise beginning and ending position.

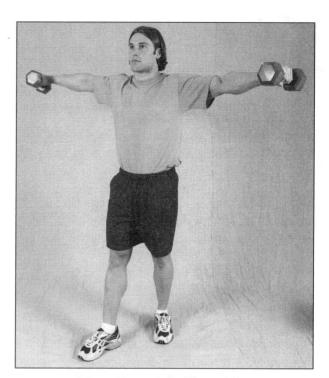

Lateral raise midpoint position.

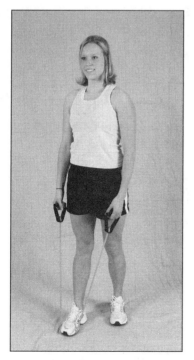

Lateral raise with tubing beginning and ending position.

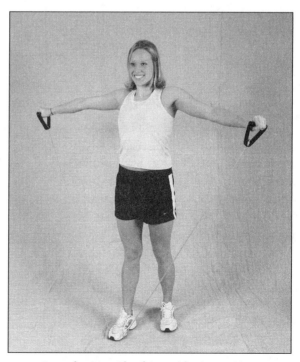

Lateral raise with tubing midpoint position.

Angled Raise: Level 1

This is an exercise that you probably won't see in any other exercise book—mainly because it emphasizes a part of your deltoid that most people ignore since you can't see it in the mirror. Well, what about those people looking at you from behind? They can see this muscle, or lack of it. If you truly want knockout shoulders, you can't afford to ignore any part of the deltoid that is visible, and the back of the shoulder is right there for everyone to see.

Preparation

1. Stand with your feet together. Hold a dumbbell in each hand. For this exercise, you will probably use a lighter weight than you normally do when working the front or middle portions of the deltoid because the back part is typically not as strong to begin with (it will be later, though).

2. Turn your hands so that your thumbs are pointing toward your legs. This is an odd way to hold a dumbbell, but you'll get used to it.

Movement

3. The angled part of this exercise comes in now. When you lift the dumbbell in the air, don't point your arm straight out in front of you or straight out to your side, but halfway in between—kind of at a diagonal to your body.

4. Keep your thumb pointed toward the floor as you lift the dumbbell to shoulder level. Slowly return it to your leg and repeat with the other arm. Alternate left- and right-side repetitions.

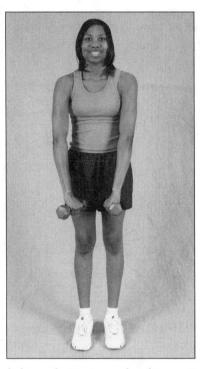

Angled raise beginning and ending position.

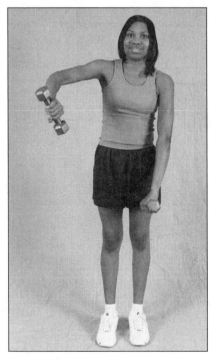

Angled raise midpoint position.

Variations

Level 1: You can do this lift with resistance tubing as well. Stand with one foot on the middle of the tubing, and hold one handle in each hand. Point your thumbs toward the floor as you lift one arm to shoulder level and back down. Alternate left and right arms. Remember to angle your lift at a diagonal to your body (not to the front or side, but somewhere in between).

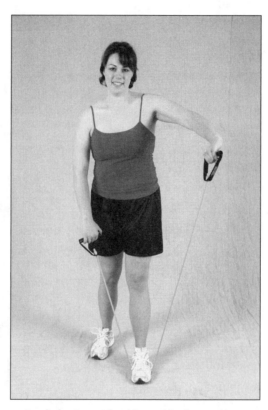

Angled raise with tubing midpoint position.

Upright Row: Level 1

Most of the "row" exercises are for the back, but this one ignores the back and focuses on the shoulders. In fact, any time you pick up something off the floor to put on a counter, get the groceries out of the trunk, or pull up your pants in the morning, you are mimicking the upright row. I call this the "pick me up" exercise because it's exactly what you do to pick up a small child. So if you don't have kids around to act as your weights (or if you do and you want to have the strength to lift them more easily), try this simple exercise to create a knockout look for your shoulders.

Preparation

1. Hold a dumbbell in each hand, palms facing your legs. Stand with your feet slightly apart for balance.

Movement

2. Imagine that there are strings tied to your elbows and someone is pulling up on the strings. Your elbows should lift up in the air, and the dumbbells should follow.

3. Bring the dumbbells right up under your chin, without actually hitting yourself (don't laugh, this actually happens). Keep the dumbbells close together. When you finish, your elbows should be higher than your wrists.

4. Slowly lower the dumbbells in front of you.

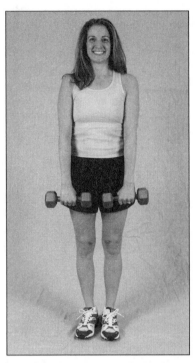

Upright row beginning and ending position.

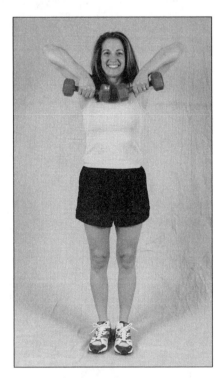

Upright row midpoint position.

Variations

Level 2: You can also do this exercise one arm at a time and work with more weight. Keep your body straight, and lift one elbow straight up in the air. Your other hand should hold a dumbbell in front of you for balance.

Level 1: Sometimes we have one arm that's stronger than the other, which will become apparent when you do this exercise. When the weaker arm gets tired, you won't be able to lift it as high as the stronger arm. To avoid this situation, use a barbell instead of dumbbells. With a barbell, the strength of both arms is combined to work together, so the stronger side can help the weaker side catch up.

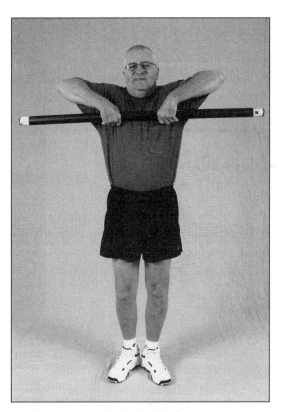

Upright row with a barbell midpoint position.

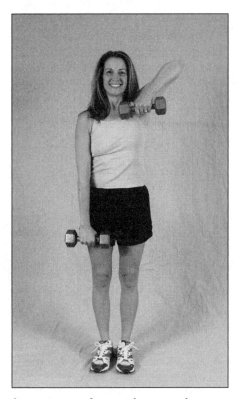

Midpoint position for upright row with one arm.

Shoulder-Press Machine: Level 1

The shoulder-press machine is a great way to work the front, middle, and back portions of your shoulders at one time. The direction the machine travels is preset, so you don't have to worry about balance or coordination; all you have to do is provide the pushing power. This exercise is done sitting down, so all your effort is focused on pushing up using the shoulders; this makes it a great isolation exercise. It's also nearly impossible to do this one wrong (unless you sit on the machine backward, which I don't advise).

Preparation

1. Adjust the seat on the machine so that when you sit down, the handles are right next to your shoulders. If the seat is too high, it will be difficult to grip the handles and probably impossible to lift. If the seat is too low, you won't experience a full range of motion, and the exercise won't be as effective.

2. There are usually two sets of handles, one set pointing at you and one set pointing out in front of you. It doesn't matter which set you use; just be sure to use the same handle on each side.

3. Sit straight in the seat. Keep your back as flat as possible during the movement. You may feel that you need to arch your back, but don't—keep it flat.

4. Place your feet flat on the floor, with a wide stance for good balance.

Movement

5. Push up with both arms until they are completely straight. The machine guides the handles, so you don't have to worry about them going the right way—there is no wrong way.

6. Slowly let your arms back down until the weight stack almost touches, and then push back up. If you allow the weight to rest, you take all the work off the shoulders and the exercise is less effective.

In the Mirror

Be sure to keep your back straight. If you can't lift the weight without arching your back, lower the weight. Arching your back hyperextends your vertebrae, a position that can lead to low-back pain.

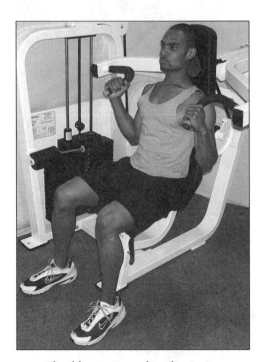

Shoulder-press machine beginning and ending position.

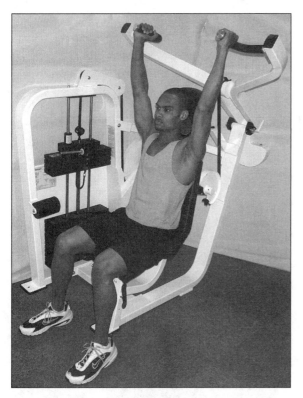

Shoulder-press machine midpoint position.

Variations

Level 2: You can isolate one shoulder with this machine by working only one arm at a time. Rest your other hand in your lap, and make sure you don't lean your body to one side while you are pushing up.

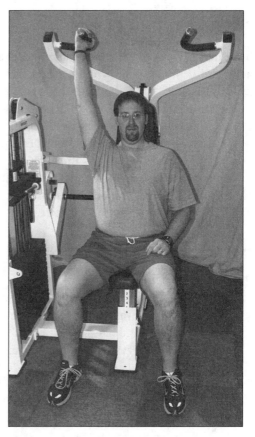

Shoulder-press machine with one hand.

Seated Press: Level 2

The seated press is similar to the shoulder-press machine, except that when you are using dumbbells or resistance tubing instead of a machine, you have to control the motion. This exercise requires a little more balance and control since your arms will go only where you tell them to go (hint: the proper direction is up). You can perform the seated press on a bench, a stability ball, or the edge of your couch, so no matter where you are, you can do this exercise.

Preparation

1. Sit on the ball or bench with your legs apart so you have a balanced stance. If you have trouble keeping your back straight— or if you tend to slouch—use a bench or chair with a back rest you can lean against.

2. Hold a dumbbell in each hand and lift them to shoulder level, placing them either in front of your shoulders or to the sides of your shoulders—whichever is more comfortable. Your hands can face toward your head or to the front; it really doesn't matter.

Movement

3. Press both dumbbells over your head at the same time. Press up until your arms are completely straight. The dumbbells should naturally move closer together and may even touch at the top. As you lift the dumbbells up and down, envision them moving along a straight line. Allowing them to sway forward or backward only wastes energy.

4. Slowly lower the dumbbells back to your shoulders.

Spot Me

If you have any back problems, forgo this exercise. Keeping your spine erect while lifting can cause great strain to your back. Also, because you are lifting a weight over your head, be sure to have a spotter to assist you.

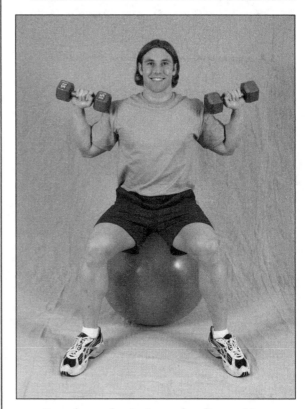

Seated press beginning and ending position.

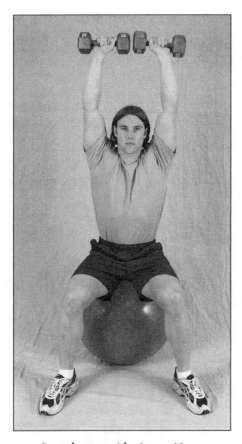

Seated press midpoint position.

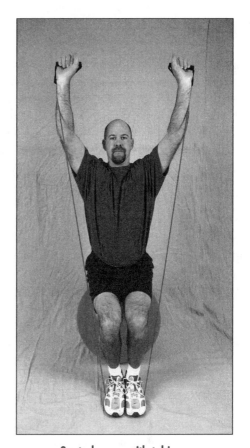

Seated press with tubing.

Variations

Level 1: If you don't have anyone to spot you, use resistance tubing instead of dumbbells. Put your feet together in front of you, and put the middle of the tubing under your feet to anchor it. Now push up with both arms at the same time. Don't forget that using resistance tubing will make it harder as you stretch out the tubing.

Military Press: Level 3

I doubt that any military group actually invented this exercise, so like most strangely named exercises, we just have to accept the term and move on. The military press is similar to the seated press, except that you use a barbell. I didn't add this as a variation to the seated press because a couple unique differences happen when you use a barbell to connect your two arms (and shoulders, in this case). The amount of weight you can lift using both shoulders together will be more than the combined weight of individual dumbbells because of a really complicated neural process that occurs somewhere in your brain (and you don't even have to think about it). This move gets your entire shoulder involved at one time and produces some of the best results I've ever seen.

Preparation

1. If possible, use a special military press bench that has an upright seat and hooks to hang the bar from. If you aren't at a gym with this equipment, you won't be able to use as much weight because you'll have to lift it from the floor to your shoulders first—which uses some energy.

2. Sit with your back flat against the seat and your feet flat on the floor in front of you. Grab hold of the bar with a shoulder-width grip (no wider).

3. Press the bar straight over your head until your arms are fully extended.

Movement

4. Slowly lower the bar in front of your head until it reaches your chin. Now push it back up.

Spot Me

There's a bar over your head, so make sure you have a spotter ready to assist you. Also, never bring the bar down behind your head: this can hurt your shoulders because of the extreme rotation involved.

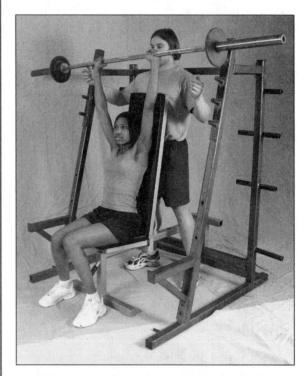

Military press beginning and ending position.

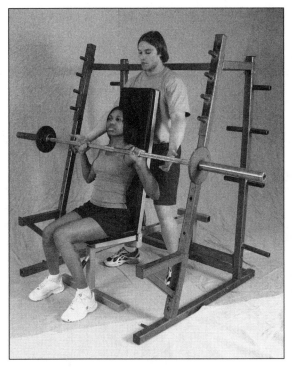

Military press midpoint position.

Variations

Level 4: You can do this exercise standing up for an even more challenging workout. Stand with one foot in front of the other for a good base of support. You may need a spotter to help you get the bar up to your shoulders to begin the exercise. From there, press it straight up over your head and lower it back to your chin.

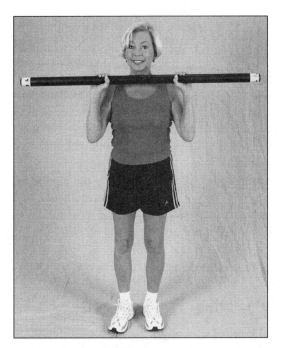

Standing military press beginning and ending position.

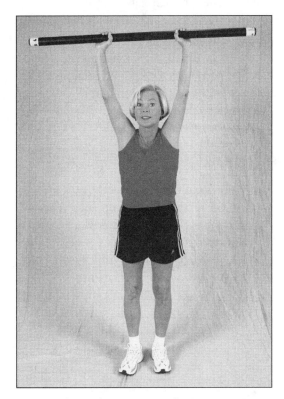

Standing military press midpoint position.

Bent-Over Lateral Raise: Level 3

Any time you bend over at the hips and lift a weight, you have to be really careful of your lower back. This exercise emphasizes the rear portion of your deltoids but also makes your lower back work to keep your upper body steady while you move. Just like the angled raise exercise, bent-over lateral raises really get into that small part on the back of your shoulder that is really noticeable, especially after you have mastered this movement and your shoulders look incredible!

Preparation

1. Stand with one foot in front of the other (it doesn't matter which is which). Hold a dumbbell in each hand.

2. Bend at the hips, making sure your back stays as straight as you can manage. Try to bend to about a 45° angle, but stop before that if you can't keep your back straight. Let your arms hang straight down under your shoulders.

Movement

3. At the same time, lift both hands up and out to the sides. Keep your arms as straight as possible. The goal is to lift your arms to the same height as your shoulders. Take care that you don't lift your whole body a bit as a way of cheating.

4. When your hands are shoulder high, slowly lower them back to the starting point. Don't let gravity do the work for you; let them down slowly and under control.

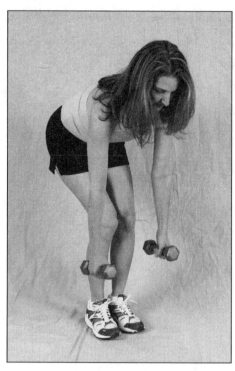

Bent-over lateral raise beginning and ending position.

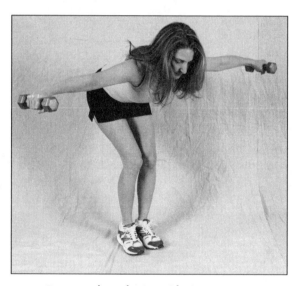

Bent-over lateral raise midpoint position.

Variations

Level 2: If you are having problems keeping your back straight and still while both arms are moving, switch to a one-arm exercise. Put one dumbbell down and use that free hand to brace against your front knee. Now complete your set on one arm; then switch to the other.

Level 4: This is another great exercise for resistance tubing; however, as the tubing stretches and becomes harder to pull, it tries to pull your body down farther. Because of this extra strain on your lower back, make sure you are ready and have mastered the dumbbell version first. Stand on the middle of the tubing, hold a handle in each hand, and pull smoothly up to shoulder height. Return the handles slowly to the starting position.

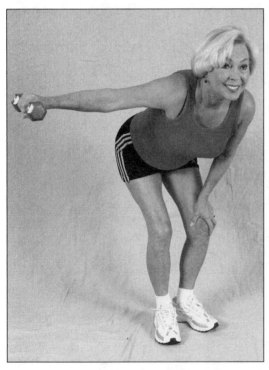

One-arm bent-over lateral raise.

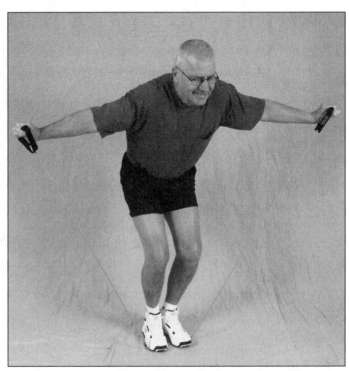

Bent-over lateral raise with tubing.

Barbell Raise: Level 3

The barbell raise works the front of the shoulders while strengthening the lower back, which acts as a stabilizer. Although both shoulders are working in synch during the barbell raise, the movement can be pretty difficult. That's because whenever you lift both arms in front of you, the weight causes your center of gravity and center of balance to move forward. To compensate for this, you have to lean back a little, which makes your lower back work very hard. If your shoulders aren't strong, your back has to work even harder. This exercise isn't meant to work your back, so you can build shoulder strength with front raises and upright rows before you attempt this exercise.

Preparation

1. Stand with your feet apart, one foot slightly behind the other. Be sure you feel steady and balanced.

2. Hold the barbell against your thighs with an overhand grip (palms facing your legs). Be sure to use a strong grip, or you risk dropping the barbell (watch out for toes). Your hands should be exactly shoulder width apart.

Movement

3. Keep your back straight, and don't let your body sway or swing back and forth. Concentrate on allowing only your shoulders to do the work.

4. With your arms straight or just slightly bent at the elbows, lift the bar in front of you until it is at shoulder height.

5. Slowly lower the bar back to your thighs.

In the Mirror

It's easy to get into a bad habit of swinging the weight into the air, using momentum instead of muscle for the movement. Concentrate on maximizing the use of your shoulders for this exercise.

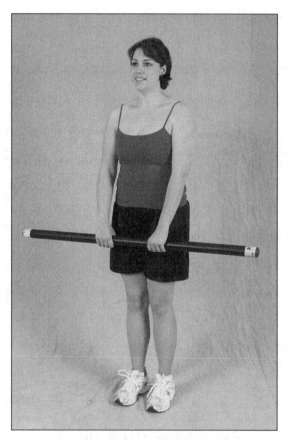

Barbell raise beginning and ending position.

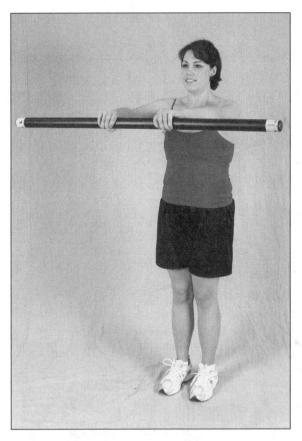

Barbell raise midpoint position.

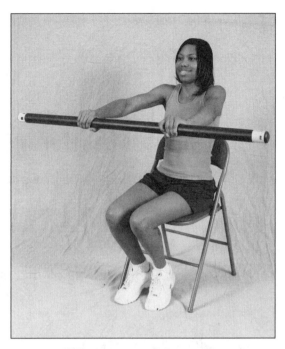

Barbell raise sitting midpoint position.

Variations

Level 2: To decrease the difficulty of this exercise and provide more support for your back, sit instead of standing. Sit on a seat with a tall back to support you. Try not to push into the back of the seat; you still need to hold your back straight all by yourself. Slowly lift the barbell to shoulder height and then lower back to your legs (it will go down to only your knees, which is fine).

In This Chapter

◆ Curling—not just a winter sport

◆ Isolating the biceps muscles

◆ Introducing EZ bars

◆ Using tubing to increase the resistance

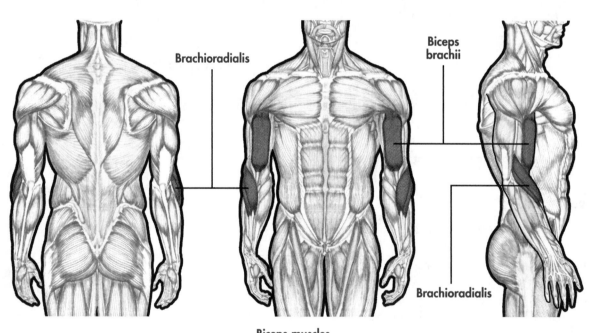

Biceps muscles.

Chapter 12

Double-Barrel Biceps

If someone walked up to you on the street and asked to "see your muscle," most people would point to and flex their biceps. Why? It may go way back to when we were kids, and flexing our biceps was the way we showed everyone how strong we were. I'm just guessing about that, but I'm pretty sure that everyone likes to have good-looking biceps. The arms are a part of the body that is almost always exposed, no matter what time of year it is. If you have knockout arms, you show them off; if you don't, you wear long sleeves all year.

The biceps are actually more than one muscle. This is a group of muscles that all work together to bend your elbow. That's their main job—bending your elbow. I've highlighted the two largest biceps muscles in the figure to the left, the biceps brachii and the brachioradialis. You will actually be able to see these muscles moving under your skin when you do these exercises (don't worry, it's not creepy or anything). This chapter includes a lot of different exercises to help you form those knockout biceps—or what I like to call the "show me your" muscle—so get to work!

Machine Curl: Level 1

The biceps curl machine is a great way to learn how to isolate and work the biceps. It's very similar to the preacher curl you'll see later in this chapter, except that the machine controls the path of movement so you don't have to. The benefit of learning this exercise using a machine instead of free weights is that the machine can move in only one direction, plus it makes both arms work together—one arm can't get ahead of the other. Bodybuilders have long used the machine curl to help them achieve a well-rounded biceps that looks good to the judges—so it should look just as good for your knockout shape.

Preparation

1. Adjust the height of the seat or the arm pad, depending on the model of bench. Your goal is to sit comfortably with your upper arms flat on the padding. If your elbows are the only part of your arms touching the pad, you are sitting too high—lower the seat. If your elbow can't touch the pad, but the top of your arms near your armpits touch it, you are sitting too low—raise the seat.

2. Grasp the handle no wider than shoulder width, with an underhand grip (palms facing up).

3. Adjust where your elbows rest on the machine so that both you and the machine pivot at the same point. There should be some kind of hinge or axis where the handle is attached to the machine. Line up your elbows with this pivot point.

Movement

4. Keep your elbows in that pivot point, and pull the bar up to your shoulders, just under your chin.

5. Slowly lower the handle back down, making sure to straighten your arms completely

before you start the next repetition. If the weight stack touches before your arms are completely straight, adjust either the seat or the alignment of your elbows.

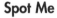

Spot Me

Don't "bounce" your arms when you lower them back down. This can strain your elbow tendons or sprain the elbow ligaments—neither of which is any fun.

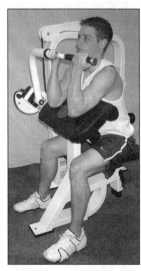

Machine curl beginning and ending position.

Machine curl midpoint position.

Preacher Curl: Level 2

You don't have to say a prayer during this exercise, but it never hurts. The preacher curl uses a special bench, similar to the machine curl, to give your arms a place to rest. This creates a more stable position for your arms than when you are holding weight. The extra support and stabilization let you focus on your biceps without worrying about keeping strict form—meaning that it's tough to mess this one up. Don't get lazy on me, though: you have to keep your arms working together to get the best benefits.

Preparation

1. Adjust the height of the seat or the arms pad, depending on the model of bench. You want to sit comfortably, with your upper arms flat on the padding. If your elbows are the only part of your arms touching the pad, you are sitting too high—lower the seat. If your elbows can't touch the pad, but the top of your arms near your armpits touch it, you are sitting too low—raise the seat.

2. Use either a regular barbell or an EZ curl bar. The EZ curl bar has become the standard on the preacher curl, so it's shown in the photos.

3. Hold the bar with a shoulder-width grip, or just a little narrower than shoulder width, using an underhand grip (palms facing up).

Movement

4. Curl the bar up to your shoulders, just under your chin.

5. Slowly lower the bar back down. Lower the weight completely until your arms are straight before you start the next repetition.

Variations

Level 1: To isolate and concentrate on one arm at a time, do the preacher curl with dumbbells. Hold one dumbbell over the bench just like you were using a barbell, and let the other hand rest in your lap.

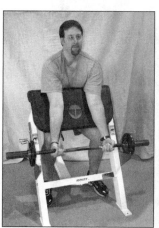
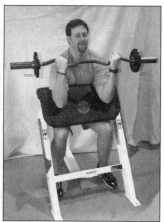
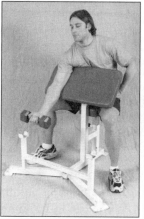
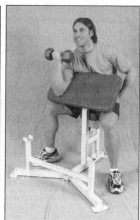

Preacher curl beginning and ending position.

Preacher curl midpoint position.

Preacher curl with dumbbell beginning and ending position.

Preacher curl with dumbbell midpoint position.

Dumbbell Curl: Level 1

I think the dumbbell curl is one of the main reasons that dumbbells were invented. Back in ancient Greek times, they probably used rocks instead of dumbbells, so we've come a long way. Dumbbell curls provide one of the best methods of isolating and applying direct resistance to the biceps. Try to do this exercise in front of the mirror, where you can see the muscle working and monitor your form.

Preparation

1. Stand with your feet apart and a dumbbell in each hand. Both dumbbells should weigh the same, even if you have one arm that's stronger. Unequal dumbbells will result in unequal results—you'll be lopsided.

2. Hold the dumbbells with an underhand grip (palms facing away from you). Let the dumbbells rest against the outside of your thighs. You arms should be completely relaxed, but not so relaxed that you drop the weight.

Movement

3. To keep from leaning back, perform the dumbbell curl with one arm at a time. (Leaning can strain your back.)

4. When lifting, keep your elbow at your side—don't let it move forward. The only part of your body that should move is your forearm and hand. Smoothly pull the dumbbell up as far as you can by bending your elbow.

5. At the top of the curl, slowly lower the dumbbell back down to rest beside your leg. Your arm should be completely straight and relaxed. Alternate arms, allowing one arm to rest while the other is working.

In the Mirror

The biggest mistake I see people making with dumbbell curls is swinging the weight. Though you may believe you're "lifting" more, you're actually letting momentum do the work for you, making the exercise less effective. Don't swing.

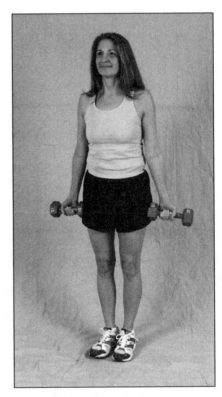

Dumbbell curl beginning and ending position.

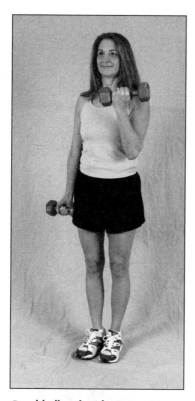

Dumbbell curl midpoint position.

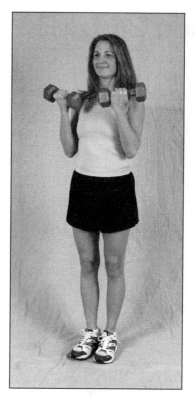

Dumbbell curl with both arms midpoint position.

Variations

Level 2: You can save time by working both arms together. The trade-off for saving time is working harder, though. To do the dumbbell curl with both arms, stand so that one foot is slightly behind you and the other foot is slightly in front of you. This will give you a wide base of support to keep you from leaning back during the curl. Pull both arms up at the same time, nice and slow; then slowly lower them back down. Do everything you can to avoid leaning back during this exercise.

Hammer Curl: Level 1

With this exercise, you hold the dumbbell as you would a hammer, and you move your arms as if you're hammering a nail—hence the name "hammer curl." Because of the way the arm is held, you won't see as much "flexing" during a hammer curl, but don't worry—you will still get a sculpted result. If you have any elbow problems (like tennis elbow) hammer curls are a good alternative to dumbbell curls, which can cause pain in a problem elbow. They put less strain on the joint, and most of my clients who do this exercise say they prefer it over dumbbell curls.

Preparation

1. Stand with your feet apart and hold a pair of dumbbells in your hands. The dumbbells should rest against the outside of your thighs—your palms should be facing your legs.

2. Keep your arms relaxed at your sides. Do not flex or bend the elbows.

Movement

3. Keep one arm at rest beside you. This exercise works one arm at a time to protect your back from unnecessary stress. Pull the other dumbbell up to your shoulder by bending your elbow. The elbow should remain at your side when you lift the dumbbell—only the forearm and hand should move.

4. Slowly let the dumbbell back down to your side, and repeat with the other arm.

Spot Me

Be sure to pay attention to where the weight is at all times. Some of my clients have actually hit themselves in the face with the dumbbell when curling it up. And as with the dumbbell curl, avoid using momentum to lift the weight—don't swing.

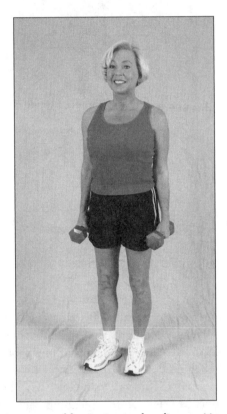

Hammer curl beginning and ending position.

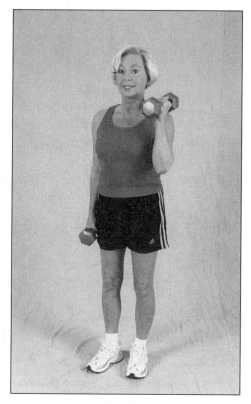

Hammer curl midpoint position.

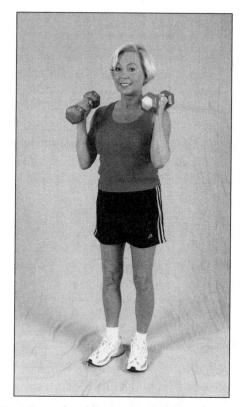

Hammer curl with both arms midpoint position.

Variations

Level 2: You can save time by working both arms at the same time. The trade-off for saving time is working harder, though. To do the dumbbell curl with both arms, stand so that one foot is slightly behind you and the other foot is slightly in front of you. This will give you a wide base of support to keep you from leaning back during the curl. Pull both arms up at the same time, nice and slow; then slowly lower them back down. Do everything you can to avoid leaning back during this exercise.

EZ Bar Curl: Level 2

If dumbbells aren't your thing and you still want to work both arms at the same time to save time, head for the barbell rack. A barbell provides the same emphasis on the biceps muscles as the dumbbell curl, but because it keeps the wrists in a locked position, the movement provides even greater benefits to both the biceps brachii and brachioradialis. An EZ bar is a type of barbell that has a wavy, bent shape to it that allows your wrists to be in a more natural position than a straight barbell allows. If you don't have an EZ bar, a regular barbell will work just fine. EZ bar curls really make your biceps flex and stand out, so do these in front of a mirror and check out your knockout results firsthand.

Preparation

1. Stand with your feet apart, with one foot slightly behind the other. You really need a solid base of support while doing this exercise because the lifting movement will make you want to lean back. Be sure to keep your back straight for proper form.

2. Hold the bar in both hands, using an underhand grip (palms facing away from you). Your grip should be about shoulder width and evenly spaced from the center or ends of the bar. Let the barbell rest against the front of your thighs.

Movement

3. Keep your body still and your elbows at your sides. Bend both elbows and curl the barbell up to your shoulders. Both sides of the barbell should reach your shoulders at the same time, so curl with a steady, balanced movement.

4. Slowly lower the barbell back down to your thighs, and relax your arms before the next repetition.

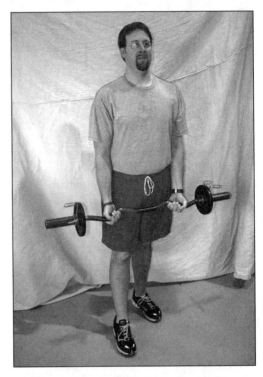

EZ bar curl beginning and ending position.

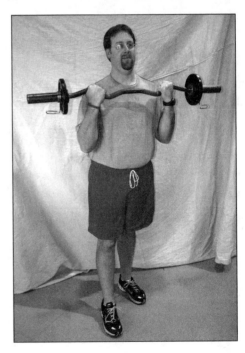

EZ bar curl midpoint position.

Low-Pulley Curl: Level 1

Pulley machines are becoming more prevalent than ever in health clubs and gyms. Many of the new styles of biceps machines use pulley systems with interchangeable handles that allow you to do different types of biceps exercises (like one-hand vs. two-hand curls). A distinct advantage of pulley machines over dumbbells, barbells, and tubing is that the resistance remains constant throughout the range of motion. With dumb-bells and barbells, there is very little resistance at the midway point of the exercise, so the low-pulley curl can give you a knockout advantage by challenging your muscle the entire time.

Preparation

1. Low-pulley machines have a number of dif-ferent handle attachments to choose from. I prefer to use the straight bar for biceps curls because it gets both arms work-ing together, which saves time. Attach a straight handle bar to the low pulley cable.

2. Grasp the handle with an underhand grip (palms facing away from you). The grip placement depends on how wide the handle is. Use a close grip that allows your hands to be at least 6 inches apart but never wider than your shoulders.

3. Let your arms relax so the bar is hanging in front of you. Step back until you are about 2 feet from the bottom pulley. Spread your feet apart, and put one foot in front of the other for good balance. When you do the low-pulley curl, you will feel as if you're being pulled forward. A good stance will prevent you from falling toward the machine.

Movement

4. Keeping your elbows at your sides, curl the bar up to your shoulders.

5. Slowly lower the bar until your arms are straight again.

In the Mirror

Really concentrate on keeping your body from leaning back or forward. Leaning may compromise the effects of the exercise and could even lead to injury.

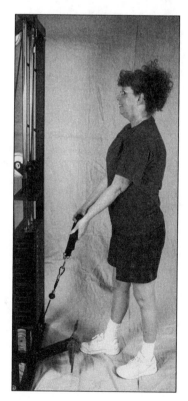

Low-pulley curl beginning and ending position.

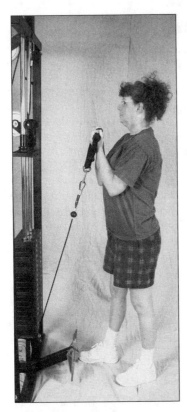

Low-pulley curl midpoint position.

Variations

Level 1: You can perform this exercise with one arm at a time. Attach a single-hand handle instead of the bar to the pulley. Stand in the same position as before, but place the hand that is not working on your hip to keep it out of the way. Complete your repetitions on one arm, and then switch to the other side.

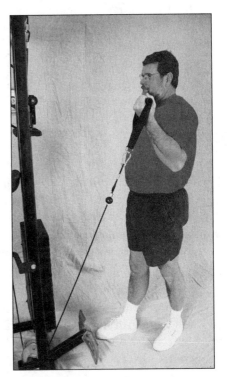

Low-pulley curl with one hand midpoint position.

Tubing Curl: Level 2

The tubing curl is effective because it becomes increasingly difficult as you perform each repetition. Unlike dumbbells and barbells that get easier near the top of the movement, or low pulleys that have the same level of difficulty throughout, tubing curls challenge the muscles more as the tubing stretches and the exercise goes on. You can adjust the resistance simply by moving the foot that anchors the tubing, and you can perform the exercise with either one or two arms at a time—you have lots of knockout ways to complete this exercise.

Preparation

1. Stand with your feet apart, one foot in front of the other.
2. Hold the ends of the tubing in each hand, using an underhand grip (palms facing up). Keep your arms relaxed and down at your sides.
3. Place the center of the tubing under your front foot. To anchor the tubing, place it under the arch of your foot—if it's too near the toe or heel, it could slip out. Place most of your body weight on the front foot.

Movement

4. To work both arms at the same time, keep your elbows at your sides and curl the tubing up to your shoulders. Remember, it will get more difficult as the tubing stretches, so keep pulling and don't give up.
5. Slowly let the tubing back down. Straighten your elbows until your arms are again relaxed at your sides.
6. If you need to make this exercise easier or harder, either use a different level of tubing or move your foot farther away from you (harder) or closer (easier).

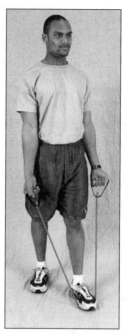 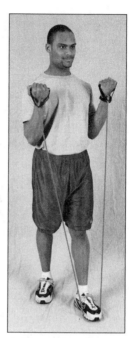

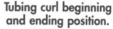

Tubing curl beginning and ending position.   Tubing curl midpoint position.

Variations

Level 2: Instead of exercising both arms at once, alternate one arm at a time or complete an entire set on one arm, followed by the other. When isolating one arm, keep holding the tubing in the other hand for support and balance.

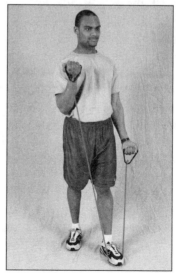

One-arm tubing curl midpoint position.

Reverse Curl: Level 2

Any time you use an overhand position with a biceps exercise (your palms face down instead of up), you make your forearms work harder because they are responsible for maintaining your grip. But how does this benefit the biceps? Many clients cannot do a full set of biceps curls because their grip is weak and they cannot hold on to the dumbbell or barbell. Overhand curls help you improve your grip while also exercising the biceps, so you really do get two exercises for the price of one.

Preparation

1. Stand with your feet apart, one foot slightly in front of the other. Hold the barbell with an overhand grip (palms facing down or toward your legs). Your grip should be evenly placed on the barbell, slightly wider than shoulder width.

2. Rest the barbell against the front of your thighs, with your arms relaxed.

Movement

3. Keep a tight grip on the barbell, and keep your elbows next to your sides. Curl the barbell up to your shoulders.

4. Slowly lower the barbell back down to rest on your thighs (maintaining a tight grip).

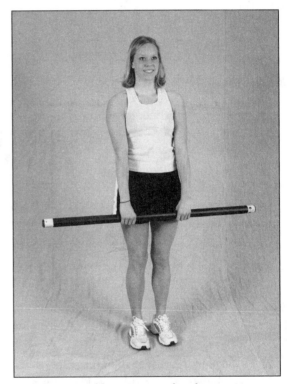

Spot Me

This exercise is designed to strengthen your forearms so you can do more biceps exercises. When your forearms become fatigued, your grip weakens. If your grip weakens, you could drop the barbell. So as soon as you get tired and fear you might drop it, your set is over. Rest a bit before you start another set.

Reverse curl beginning and ending position.

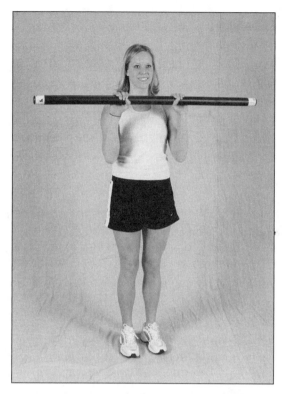

Reverse curl midpoint position.

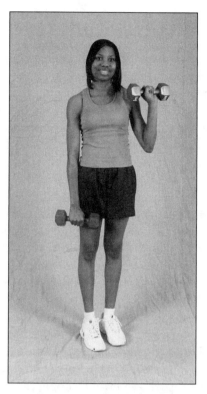

One-arm reverse curl with
dumbbells midpoint position.

Variations

Level 1: You can do this exercise with dumbbells, if you like. Use the same movement, but
alternate or work one arm at a time. That way,
you can concentrate on the grip even more.

Concentration Curl: Level 2

Concentration curls get their name because you have to concentrate on completing a set with just one arm at a time while keeping the strictest of form. A concentration curl is a bit more difficult than other dumbbell curls because you are concentrating all your effort on one little muscle group that's being worked repeatedly without any rest. The upside is that this exercise makes the biceps work more and the results often show it. It's also an ideal exercise for helping a weaker arm catch up to a stronger one. Because you are working one arm at a time, you can do a few extra reps or an extra set for the weaker arm until both arms have equal strength.

Preparation

1. Sit on the end of a bench, or on a stool, chair, or stability ball. Spread your feet wide apart—you will be doing this exercise between your legs.

2. Place your left hand on your left knee for support while you work your right arm (switch this to work your left arm).

3. Hold the dumbbell with an underhand grip (palm facing away from you), and let the dumbbell hang down inside your leg.

4. Bend at the waist—keeping your back straight—and let your elbow rest against the inside of your leg, right next to your knee.

Movement

5. Brace your elbow against your leg, bend your elbow, and curl the weight up toward your shoulder. Don't let the dumbbell hit you in the face.

6. Slowly lower the dumbbell until the arm is completely straight; then repeat until you finish the set.

In the Mirror

You might feel like you need to lean back or to the side to help you curl when you start getting tired. Don't do this—be sure to keep your back straight during the whole exercise. You want to focus your effort on the biceps muscles, and leaning is a form of cheating that will decrease your results. The only part of your body that should be moving is your forearm and hand.

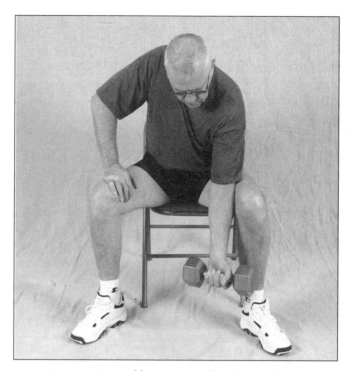

Concentration curl beginning and ending position.

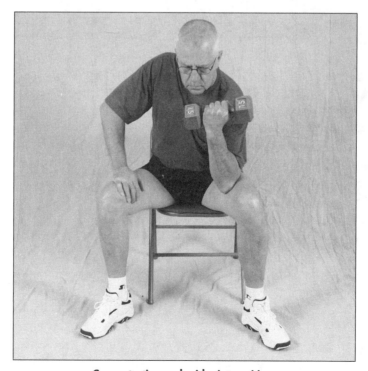

Concentration curl midpoint position.

In This Chapter

- ◆ Flappy arm syndrome
- ◆ Kickbacks are a good thing
- ◆ Pushing up and down
- ◆ How the French do it

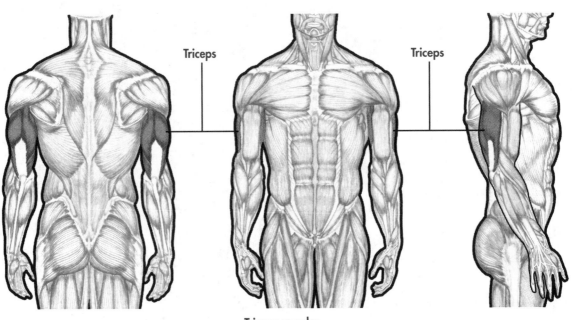

Triceps muscles.

You Gotta Try These Triceps

When I was preparing to write this book, I had a couple clients tell me that the triceps chapter should come at the very beginning because that is an area a lot of women want to work on. I agree that it is a problem area for a lot of people suffering from the "flappy arm syndrome," but I don't think any one muscle group is that much more important than any other muscle group—they all have to be worked.

That being said, the triceps do a lot of work during other exercises, especially during chest exercises. Any time you straighten your arm in a pushing movement, the triceps are working. During chest exercises, they are called assistant muscles. In this chapter, we focus on how to work the triceps in isolation and turn any "flappy arms" into well-sculpted knockout arms.

Kickback: Level 1

The kickback is a staple of triceps exercises. This exercise allows you to isolate each arm independently, giving each set of triceps muscles lots of attention. In a standing position, all you have to do to straighten your elbow is just relax your arm; however, the kickback puts you in a position in which relaxing your arm bends the elbow so you have to work to straighten it. I highly suggest that you do this one in front of a mirror because you can keep an eye on proper form—and the definition of your sculpted knockout muscles.

Preparation

1. To work your left arm, place your right hand and knee on the exercise bench (or the edge of your bed). Hold the dumbbell in your left hand, with your palm facing your body. Your left foot should be on the floor. Keep your back flat and your shoulders parallel to the floor.

2. Lift your left elbow until your upper arm is parallel to the floor. Your elbow should be at about your side. If you get tired and your elbow drops from this position, the effectiveness of this exercise drops considerably, so keep your elbow high.

Movement

3. Extend your arm until it's completely straight and the dumbbell is back by your hips.

4. Slowly lower the dumbbell back to the starting point. Don't let the dumbbell "swing" back down or pass the starting point.

5. When you complete a set on the left side, turn around, place your left hand and knee on the bench, hold the dumbbell in your right hand, and complete a set for your right arm.

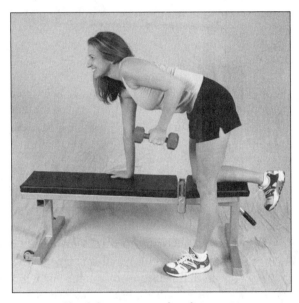

Kickback beginning and ending position.

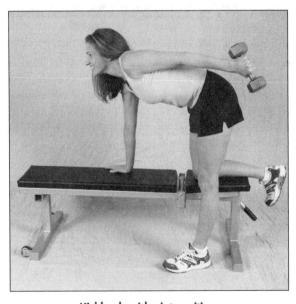

Kickback midpoint position.

Variations

Level 2: For more resistance and a larger range of motion, use resistance tubing instead of dumbbells. Anchor your tubing to a doorway or machine in front of you about waist high. Hold the other handle in one hand. Instead of starting with the weight hanging down, you start with the your hand near your shoulder; the tubing will pull you into this position. Extend your hand all the way back toward your hips, and slowly return to the starting position.

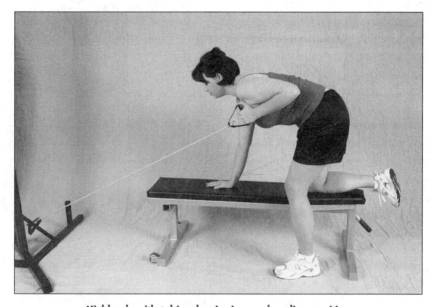

Kickback with tubing beginning and ending position.

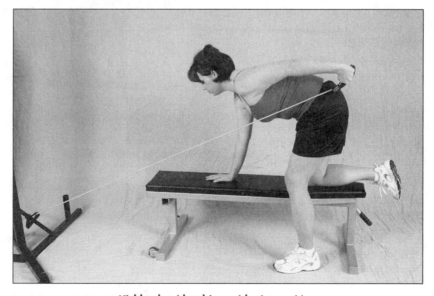

Kickback with tubing midpoint position.

Overhead Press: Level 1

The overhead press may seem a bit awkward at first, but when you get a few sets under your belt, you're sure to be comfortable with it. The advantage of this exercise is that the triceps start in a slightly stretched position, so they have to work even harder to overcome the resistance. Second, this is the position in which the "flappy arm syndrome" is most noticeable, so working it here will allow you to see the results fast.

Preparation

1. Sit on an exercise bench or on the edge of a chair (be sure the chair has a short back).

2. Hold a dumbbell in one hand, but instead of holding on to the handle, cup one end of the dumbbell in your palm so you're holding the dumbbell the long way. Your thumb should be on one side of the handle, and your fingers should be on the other. See the photo for clarification.

3. To work your right arm, hold the dumbbell straight up in the air slightly behind your head (don't hold it over your head, in case you drop it). Place your other hand on your knee for support. Keep your back straight at all times.

Movement

4. Bend your elbow and lower the dumbbell behind your head. Keep your elbow pointed up in the air at all times. Lower the dumbbell behind you as far as your elbow will bend.

5. Straighten your arm and lift the dumbbell back up.

6. After a set on one side, switch arms and work the other side.

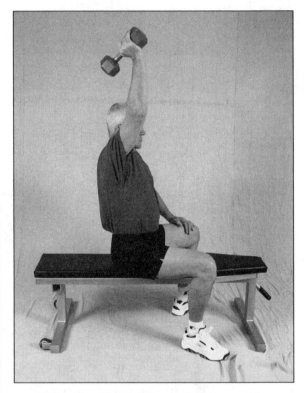

Overhead press beginning and ending position.

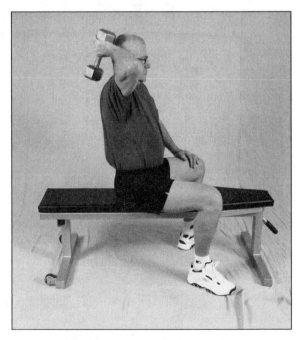

Overhead press midpoint position.

Variations

Level 1: If the dumbbell becomes too heavy or big to safely hold in one hand, grip it with both hands to work both triceps at once. Concentrate on keeping your back as straight as possible when doing this variation because you won't have one hand on your knee for support; your back has to do all the work to keep you straight.

Level 1: Use resistance tubing instead of a dumbbell. Hold one handle of the tubing over your head. Let the tubing hang down behind your back. Reach around your back with your free hand and grab hold of the tubing. This hand is now the tubing anchor. You can adjust how hard it is to extend your hand by moving the lower hand up or down the tubing.

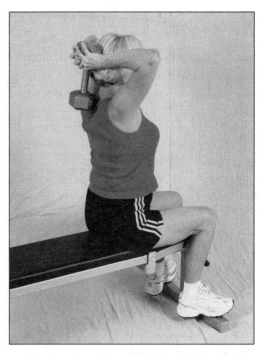

Overhead press with two hands midpoint position.

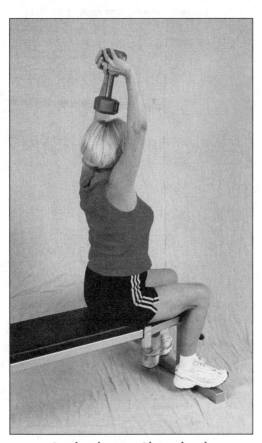

Overhead press with two hands beginning and ending position.

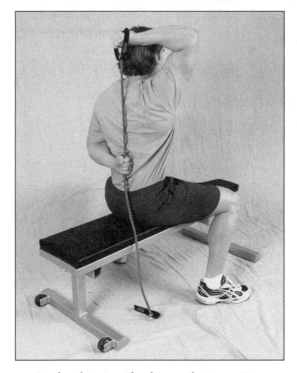

Overhead press with tubing midpoint position.

Lying Press: Level 1

It may look like the lying press is just a more relaxed version of the overhead press, but it's actually quite different. In the lying position, the triceps aren't stretched out as much in the starting position, so you can use more weight with this exercise. More weight, or resistance, equals more results. Since you will have a weight over your head during parts of this exercise, it's a good idea to have a spotter handy.

Preparation

1. Lie on your back on an exercise bench or aerobics step. Place your feet flat on the floor for support and balance.
2. Hold a dumbbell in one hand. Keep your thumb wrapped around the handle to maintain a strong grip.
3. Hold the dumbbell over your chest and shoulders. Place your other hand on your arm just below your elbow, using it to steady and support your lifting arm.

Movement

4. Bend your elbow and slowly lower the dumbbell until it's just beside your head at ear level. Your supporting hand should keep your elbow from moving.
5. Straighten your arm using your triceps, raising the dumbbell back to the starting position. After a set on one side, switch arms and do another set.

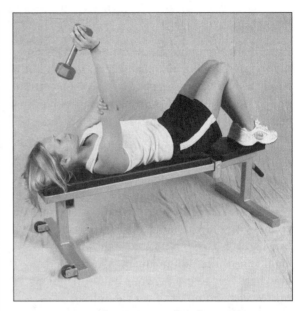

Lying press beginning and ending position.

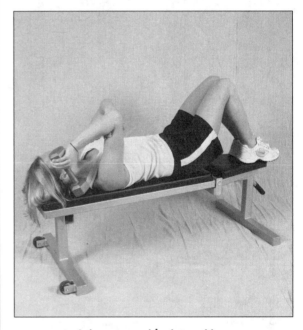

Lying press midpoint position.

Variations

Level 2: You can save some time if you use both arms at the same time. This is a little more advanced because you won't have the free arm to help support the working arm. Hold a dumbbell in each hand and move both arms up and down together. Make sure you have a spotter for this one.

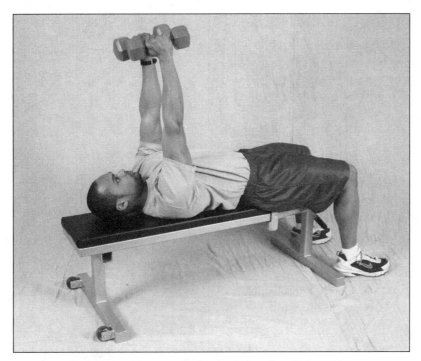

Lying press with two arms beginning and ending position.

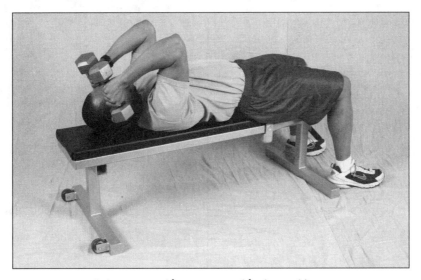

Lying press with two arms midpoint position.

French Curl: Level 3

This exercise is one of the only effective methods of working the triceps with a barbell. Do not attempt it unless you have a reasonable amount of strength in your triceps already; this is an advanced exercise. The French curl is so effective because it stretches the triceps at the midway point, so the muscles have to work harder to overcome both this extra stretch and the weight of the barbell. Because it's more challenging, it's also highly effective in creating a knockout look.

Preparation

1. Lie on your back on an exercise bench or aerobics step. Place both feet flat on the ground for support and stability.

2. Hold the barbell with a shoulder-width grip, palms facing up. Keep your thumbs wrapped around the bar to prevent it from slipping out of your hands. Hold the barbell straight up over your chest and shoulders.

Movement

3. Keeping your elbows in the starting position and your upper arms perpendicular to the floor, slowly bend your elbows and lower the barbell toward the top of your head. Don't let the bar touch your head.

4. When the bar is almost touching the top of your head (your spotter will tell you when this occurs) use the triceps to straighten your arms, pushing the barbell back up to the starting point.

Spot Me

This exercise has a nickname among those who do it frequently— the "skull-crusher." That's because of the dangers of performing this exercise without a spotter. If you don't have a spotter, try one of the other triceps exercises outlined in this chapter.

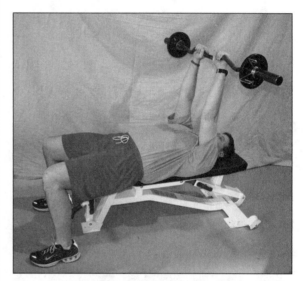

French curl beginning and ending position.

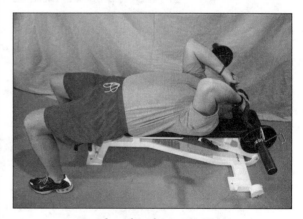

French curl midpoint position.

Variations

Level 3: If you don't have a barbell handy, use a single dumbbell. Hold the dumbbell in both hands, with either both hands on the handle or one hand on each end of the dumbbell. Perform the rest of the exercise exactly the same as with the barbell.

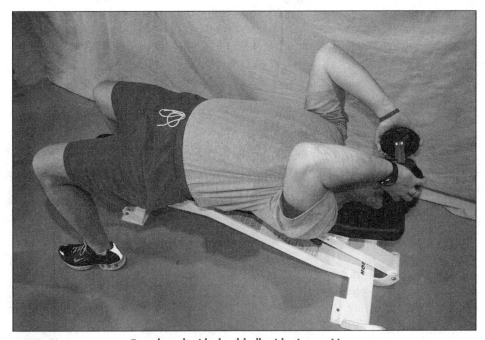

French curl with dumbbell midpoint position.

Standing Pushdown: Level 1

The standing pushdown simulates the motion of getting up from a chair or out of the swimming pool, or closing your suitcase when it's too full. The standing pushdown exercise provides a full range of motion, and you won't have to concentrate on balancing or holding on to a barbell or dumbbell. Instead, you can relax your grip a bit and really focus your effort on working your triceps, without expending extra energy hanging on to a weight.

Preparation

1. Attach a straight handle or a triceps v-handle to a high pulley cable. You can use many different types of handles for this exercise, but the straight or triceps v-handle enables the best form. Some bodybuilders like to use a handle made of rope, but that just makes your forearms work harder—which is not the focus of this exercise.

2. Grasp the handle with one hand on each side of the cable, evenly spaced from the middle to prevent tilting. Use an overhand grip (palms facing down). Keep your grip relaxed, and focus on pushing down with the flat part of your palms.

3. Stand as close to the cable as possible without getting under it. If you find that the handle is swinging away from you during the exercise, you are too close—back up. Keep your feet apart, with one foot in front of the other for good balance.

4. Gripping the handle, bend your elbows so that your hands come as close to your shoulders as possible. This is your starting position, and it is the highest point that your hands will be positioned during the exercise.

Movement

5. Keeping your elbows at your sides, push down with both arms until your elbows are straight.

6. Slowly let the elbows bend and bring the handle back up to the starting position. Keep your elbows at your sides throughout this exercise. If your elbows start to move forward, don't raise your hands any higher.

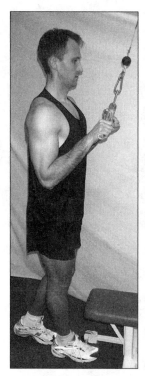 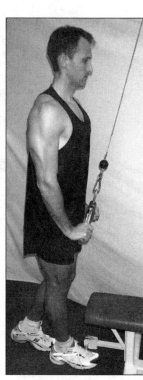

Standing pushdown beginning and ending position.

Standing pushdown midpoint position.

Variations

Level 1: You can do this exercise one arm at a time by using a single-handed attachment. This allows you to isolate each arm by itself and can help you overcome strength imbalances between arms.

Level 2: Instead of using a high-pulley cable machine, use resistance tubing. Attach the tubing to the top of a door, or loop it over the top of a machine. Hold one handle in each hand and perform the exercise exactly the same as described for the cable. If there is too much slack in the tubing, wrap it around your hands a couple times. Remember that since you are using tubing, the exercise will get harder as the tubing stretches near the midpoint.

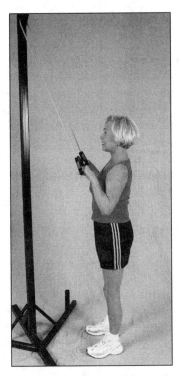

Standing pushdown with tubing beginning and ending position.

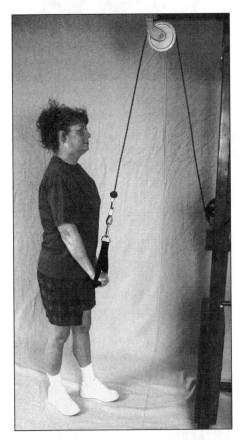

One-hand standing pushdown midpoint position.

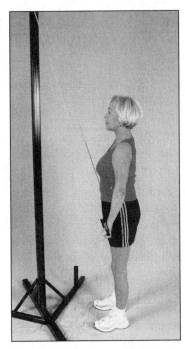

Standing pushdown with tubing midpoint position.

Triceps-Press Machine: Level 1

This form of the triceps-press machine has become the norm for most equipment brands. It is basically the same exercise as the barbell French curl, except that you are sitting instead of lying, and there is no way the bar can land on your head (so you don't need a spotter). With an established range of motion and no chance of dropping a barbell, it's a safe and effective method of working the triceps.

Preparation

1. Adjust the height of the seat so that when you put your arms on the pad, your elbows and a large portion of your upper arms are touching the pad. If only your elbows are touching the pad, you are seated too high. If your elbows aren't touching the pad, you're seated too low.

2. Slide forward or back in the seat until your elbows line up with the pivot point of the machine. The pivot point is where the handles attach to the axis of the machine—it's usually explained on the machine's instruction card or is painted a different color than the machine. Line up your elbows with the pivot point so that you are working *with* the machine, not against it.

3. You don't need to use the back support pad if you can maintain a straight seated position, but if it's more comfortable, adjust the pad so that it just touches your back.

4. Place your feet flat on the floor in front of you. Grasp the handles, one in each hand, and pivot the handle arm back toward you. It may feel a bit awkward at first, but that will pass when you get the hang of the exercise.

Movement

5. Keep your elbows in place and push against the handles until your arms are completely straight.

6. Slowly bend your elbows back up to return the handles to the start position. This is the most intense part of the exercise because you really have to work your triceps to keep your elbows from rising off the pad. You'll probably feel your triceps muscles "burn" with the effort.

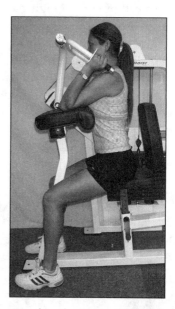

Triceps-press machine beginning and ending position.

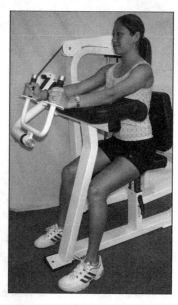

Triceps-press machine midpoint position.

Seated Dips: Level 2

Any time you push yourself out of a chair or off the couch, you are actually doing a small version of the seated dip. The great thing about the seated dip exercise is that it requires no special equipment: you can use a chair, a bench, a stool, an aerobics step, or your couch for this exercise. That also means you'll never have an excuse for skipping it!

Preparation

1. Find a flat bench, a chair, an aerobics step, or even your couch. Whatever you choose to use, make sure that it is stable enough that it won't tip over or slide when you push down on the edge of it.
2. Sit on the edge of the bench with your hands on the bench right at your sides, with your fingers pointing toward your feet.
3. Holding yourself up by your arms, scoot your butt off the edge of the bench and slide your feet out in front of you.

Movement

4. Slowly let your elbows and hips bend, as if you were going to sit down on the floor. Lower yourself until your shoulders are at the same level as your elbows and your upper arms are parallel with the floor. If you end up sitting on the floor, you've gone too low—or your bench isn't high enough.
5. Push on your hands to push yourself back to the starting position.

Spot Me

If you've ever dislocated your shoulder, or if you experience any shoulder pain while performing this exercise, do not continue. Try one of the other triceps exercises in this chapter as an alternative.

Variations

Level 2: You are only pushing against the weight of your body, so the resistance doesn't get much more challenging—unless we rearrange your body and add more external weight. Place your feet on a bench or chair of the same height as you are using for your hands. Have a spotter place a weight plate on your thighs when you are in the starting position. Start light and add weight as you can handle it. Complete the movement as described previously.

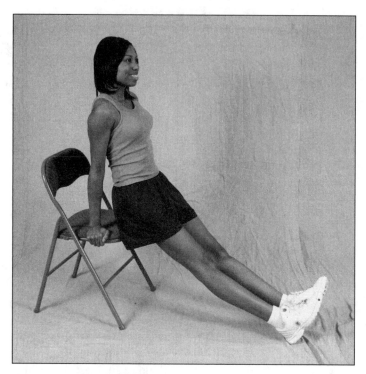

Seated dip beginning and ending position.

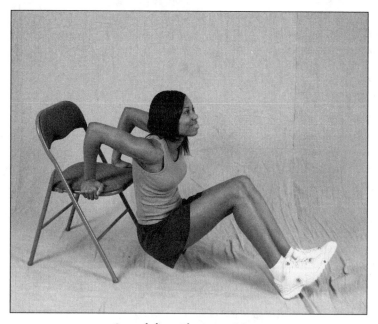

Seated dip midpoint position.

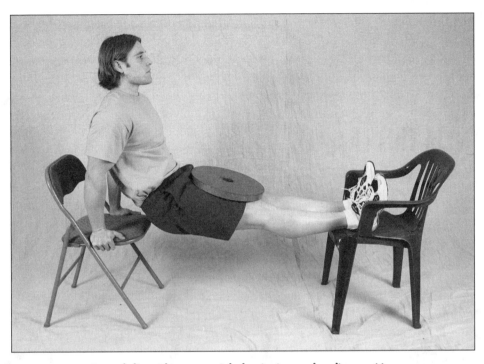

Seated dip with extra weight beginning and ending position.

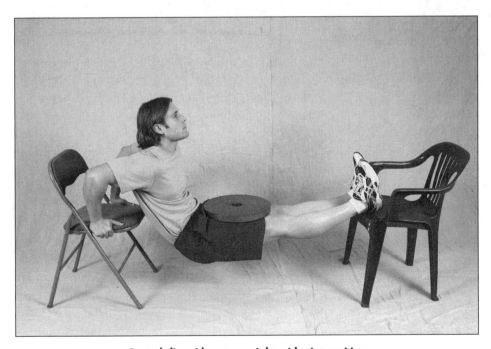

Seated dip with extra weight midpoint position.

In This Chapter

- ◆ Working to the maximus
- ◆ It started with Jane Fonda
- ◆ Squeeze the buns
- ◆ Kick like a donkey

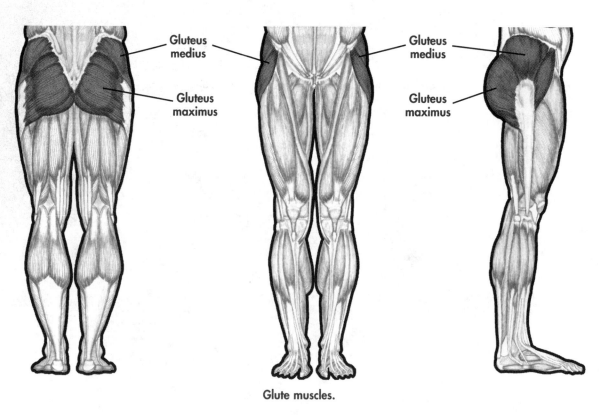

Gluteus medius

Gluteus maximus

Gluteus medius

Gluteus maximus

Glute muscles.

Chapter 14

Don't Leave This Behind

To be brutally honest, I've never heard anyone say they don't care what their backside looks like. Unfortunately, the glutes and hips are two areas where a lot of people store excess fat. As luck would have it, we can work both areas at the same time using the same exercises. The two large glute muscles, the gluteus maximus and medius, are the powerhouse muscles of your butt. These are muscles that have a lot of endurance properties, which means that no matter how much or how hard you work them, they won't get bigger—they'll just get firmer. This is totally different from most other muscles that do get bigger with exercise. Some people may disagree with me on this, but just look at the professional bodybuilders who work as hard as they can on their butts—the muscles end up small and firm, not big and cushy. That's my point!

Any time you walk, jump, climb stairs, or move your leg in just about any way you can think of, your glutes are involved. This chapter focuses on the exercises that isolate and emphasize these muscles. The thing I like the most about working the glutes is the feeling that reminds you they are working: these muscles have lots of nerve endings that send screaming messages to your brain to let you know they are working hard (hence the term "a pain in my butt").

Superman Squeeze: Level 1

Superman flies through the air with the greatest of ease while wearing tights that don't hide anything—especially his glutes. You won't be able to fly after this exercise, but your backside will definitely be ready to put on tights. This is a small-movement exercise, so don't let the ease of this one fool you. Some of the best exercises come in the smallest packages.

Preparation

1. Lie on your stomach on the floor, using either a carpeted surface or an exercise mat (a hard floor just isn't any fun).

2. Stretch out your arms in front of you, and point your toes behind you. Keep your palms flat on the floor and the tips of your toes touching the floor.

Movement

3. Lift one leg off the floor as high as you can without lifting your hips or rolling to one side. Really focus on squeezing the butt muscles as you lift.

4. Slowly lower that foot back to the floor and repeat the lift until you have finished your set with that leg. Now do a set for the other leg.

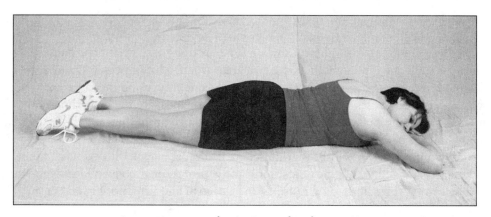

Superman squeeze beginning and ending position.

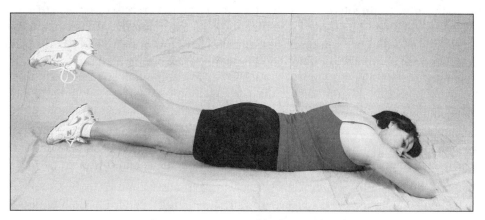

Superman squeeze midpoint position.

Variations

Level 2: You'll probably outgrow the normal Superman squeeze really fast, so here is a way to make it even more challenging. Lie over a stability ball, with the top of the ball just at your hips. Keep your hands on the floor for balance and your feet together behind you. Lift both feet off the floor at the same time as high as possible. Slowly lower them back down and repeat again. This "double lift" saves time and makes both sets of glutes muscles work in unison for a great knockout look.

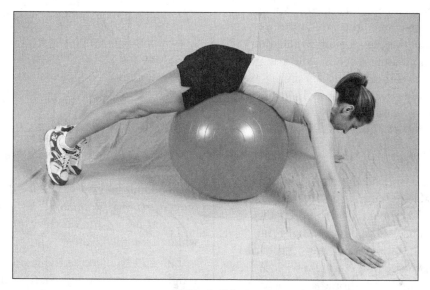

Superman squeeze on a stability ball beginning and ending position.

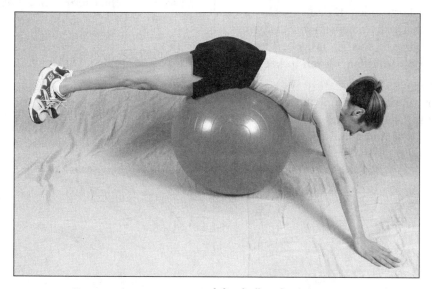

Superman squeeze on a stability ball midpoint position.

Lying Leg Lift: Level 1

Some people call this the Jane Fonda exercise because she made it popular back in the 1970s. Since then, its popularity has dropped as equipment manufacturers have produced big machines that do the same thing. I still believe that if you can work a muscle using your own weight as resistance you don't need to spend thousands on a machine. You can do this exercise (and most of the exercises in this chapter) anywhere, without a big machine, and still get knockout results. Although this is a simple exercise, it is seriously effective. You'll discover that when you start to feel the burn.

Preparation

1. Lie on your side on the floor (it's more comfortable if you have an exercise mat or a carpeted surface). Position your bottom arm (the one on the floor) straight out over your head, and rest your head it. Do not prop yourself on your elbow. Your free hand (the top hand) should rest on your hip or waist (not on the floor).

2. Bend your bottom leg (the one on the floor) so that your knee is in front of your body and your foot is behind you. This will provide a solid foundation to keep you from rolling.

3. Hold your upper leg completely straight, just off the ground. Relax your foot (it doesn't help to point your toe, like some people think).

Movement

4. Slowly lift your top leg into the air as far as you can. Make sure you don't "throw" your leg up in the air to use momentum instead of muscle—that doesn't help you in any way. Now lower your leg back to the ground, stopping just before you make contact—don't let the top leg touch the ground or your lower leg.

5. When you complete a set on this leg, roll over and work the other leg.

Variations

Level 1: You can increase the intensity by shortening the movement and speeding it up a bit. Instead of lifting your leg as high as you can, lift it only about halfway up. Since this is a smaller movement, you compensate by going faster. Lift your leg up and down as quickly as you can while staying in control.

Level 2: To increase the resistance, add ankle weights to your top leg. Start with a weight of about 1 to 2 pounds, and continue to increase the weight as the exercise becomes easier.

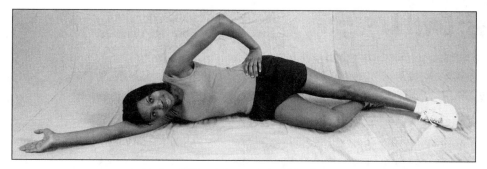

Lying leg lift beginning and ending position.

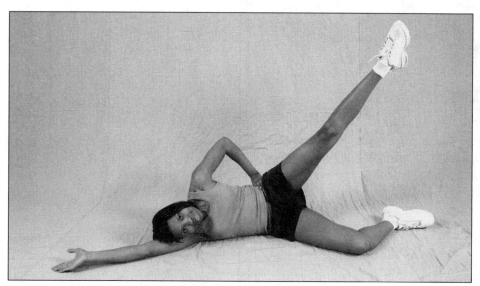

Lying leg lift midpoint position.

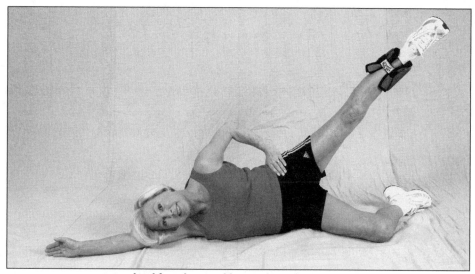

Lying leg lift with an ankle weight midpoint position.

Stomps: Level 1

The stomp exercise is similar to the lying leg lift, but it makes you use the glute muscles in a different range of motion and use a lot more control. The glute muscles work in a very large area that covers their entire range of motion, but they do not get any rest until the set is complete. This technique is known as increasing the "time under tension." The longer a muscle works continuously, the more endurance it builds. The glute muscles have a lot of endurance already, so we just pile on a little more so that knockout vibe comes calling.

Preparation

1. Lie on your side on the floor (it's more comfortable if you have an exercise mat or a carpeted surface). Position your bottom arm (the one on the floor) straight out over your head, and rest your head on it. Do not prop yourself on your elbow. Your free hand (the top hand) should rest on your hip or waist.

2. Bend your bottom leg (the one on the floor) so that your knee is in front of your body and your foot is behind you. This will provide a solid foundation to keep you from rolling.

3. Hold your upper leg completely straight, just off the ground.

Movement

4. Bring your knee up toward your chest as far as you can.

5. Immediately press it back down straight in a stomping motion (pretend a big gross bug is down there and you want to squish it). Repeat pulling and pushing the knee away from you until your set is complete.

6. When one leg is finished, roll over and work the other leg.

Variations

Level 2: Add more resistance by wearing an ankle weight. Start with 1 to 2 pounds, and increase the weight as you can handle the resistance and still finish your set.

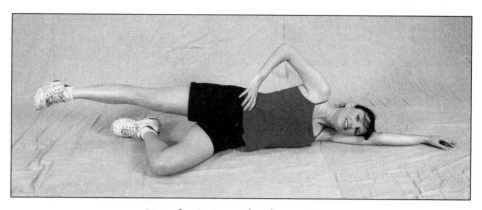

Stomp beginning and ending position.

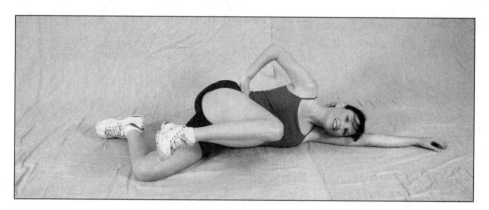

Stomp midpoint position.

Donkey Kick: Level 1

The donkey kick is one exercise that actually lives up to its name—the movement looks like a donkey kicking. Another type of leg lift, this movement focuses even more narrowly on your gluteus maximus (lower butt and "saddlebag" area). Besides delivering the obvious sculpting benefits, this exercise helps you gain strength to do traditional leg lifts even more effectively.

Preparation

1. Kneel on your hands and knees, using either a carpeted surface or an exercise mat for cushioning.

2. Place your hands directly under your shoulders and your knees directly under your hips. Keep your back flat and your head down (don't look up, to the side, or back at your legs).

Movement

3. Choose which leg you want to work first. Keep your knee bent and push the sole of your foot toward the ceiling. Move your leg back and up in the air in a smooth, slow, controlled movement (don't allow momentum to do the work).

4. Bring your leg back down toward the ground, but don't let it touch bottom. Immediately begin another repetition until your set is complete.

5. When you have finished with one leg, you'll need to rest a moment before you work the other leg. The leg you just worked has to recover before it can support your body weight.

Spot Me

Be sure to keep your back as straight as possible while your leg is moving so you don't twist and injure your spine. Your hips may swivel a bit, but your back should remain still.

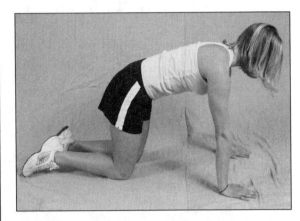

Donkey kick beginning and ending position.

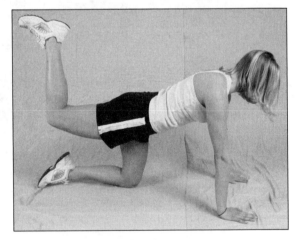

Donkey kick midpoint position.

Variations

Level 2: For more intensity, add an ankle weight. Begin with a 1- or 2-pound weight, and move up as the set becomes easier.

Level 2: To add some more range of motion, at the top of the kick, straighten your leg like you are trying to touch the ceiling.

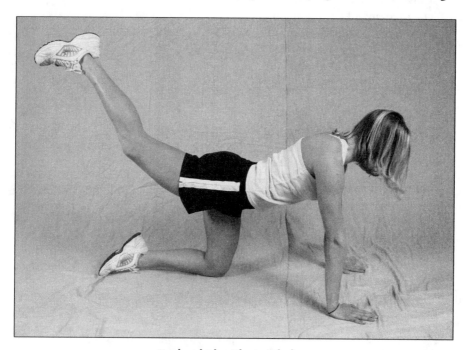

Donkey kick with straight leg.

Standing Lateral Lift: Level 2

You'll notice that this exercise is just like the lying leg lift, except that you are standing. The standing lateral lift uses a low-pulley machine to add more resistance than an ankle weight can. In addition, that resistance is always constant, whereas the resistance from an ankle weight actually decreases as you lift it higher and your leg becomes more vertical. The result is a higher level of knockout results when you're done.

Preparation

1. Attach the ankle strap to the cable from the low-pulley machine and to your leg.
2. Select the weight you are going to use from the stack, making sure the selector pin is pushed all the way in.
3. Stand so that the leg you are going to work first (the one attached to the cable/tubing) is farthest from the anchor (see photos for clarification).
4. Hold on to something stable with one hand for support. Place the other hand on your hip.

Movement

5. Keep your body as straight as possible while you lift the working leg directly out to your side as far as you can. Really concentrate on squeezing your glute muscles as you lift your leg.
6. Slowly bring your leg back under you, and repeat until your set is done. Now switch legs and do another set.

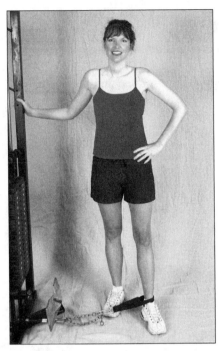

Beginning and ending position for standing lateral lift.

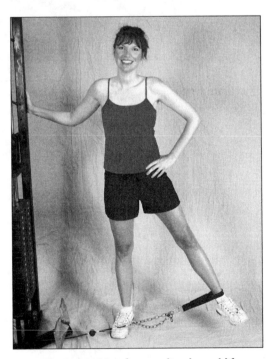

Midpoint position for standing lateral lift.

Variations

Level 3: You can make this exercise more challenging by using resistance tubing instead of a low-pulley machine. Resistance tubing requires more effort as you lift your leg farther to your side. The farther your leg is away from your body, the weaker it naturally is, so this variation focuses more effort on your weakest part in the exercise. You can either hook one handle over your toes, or wrap the tubing around your ankle and foot, and then anchor the other end around something heavy that you can't pull over. As you lift your leg to the side, keep it in constant motion and in control; don't try to "throw" it out to the side to get it higher.

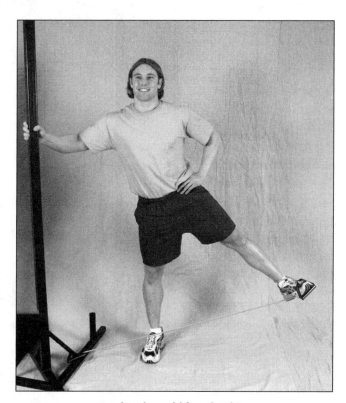

Standing lateral lift with tubing.

Standing Pushback: Level 2

The standing pushback is actually a movement called hip extension. Hip extension is the last little bit of movement you can perform with your leg from a standing position. This is just like the Superman squeeze, except that you work against a weight resistance instead of gravity. The low-pulley machine is the best for this exercise because it keeps the resistance equal through the entire motion.

Preparation

1. Attach an ankle strap to the low-pulley machine and to one leg.

2. Stand facing the weight stack. Choose the weight you want to use, and make sure the selector pin is pushed all the way in.

3. Hold on to the machine with both hands for support. Step back a bit to put some resistance on the glutes at the starting point. Shift your weight onto your support leg.

Movement

4. Keeping your leg straight, push it back as far as possible while really focusing on squeezing your glutes.

5. Slowly bring your leg back under you and repeat until you have finished your set; then transfer the ankle strap to the other leg and complete another set.

In the Mirror

It may be tempting to lean forward to try to get more extension; however, leaning forward actually decreases the effectiveness of the exercise. Keep your body as straight as possible.

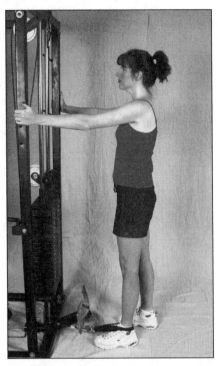

Standing pushback beginning and ending position.

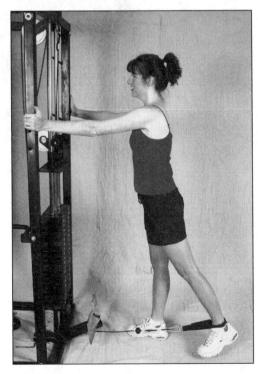

Standing pushback midpoint position.

Glute-Press Machine

The glute-press machine mimics the donkey kick exercise, except that it offers the opportunity to add resistance to really make those glutes work. This is also a good alternative if you have knee problems and you find that supporting your body weight on one knee during donkey kicks is uncomfortable.

Preparation

1. Begin by adjusting a couple of the machine's features: the height of the pad that you'll rest your elbows on, and the height of the pad you'll rest your chest on. Set both of these at a comfortable position that matches your body height. Don't hunch over the machine with pads that are too low.

2. Place one foot on the platform and one on the floor to support you. Place your platform foot flat in the middle of the platform so neither the toes nor the heels are hanging off.

3. Select the weight you want to use—be sure the selector pin is all the way in.

Movement

4. Push back with the foot on the platform as far as possible. You won't be able to completely straighten your leg because of the way the machine is designed.

5. Slowly lower the platform back to the starting position, but stop just before the weight stack comes to rest. This allows you to keep some pressure on the muscle and helps you work it more effectively.

6. Complete a set on one leg; then switch to the other.

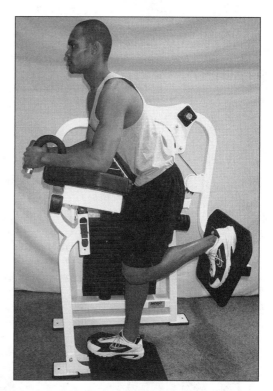

Glute-press machine beginning and ending position.

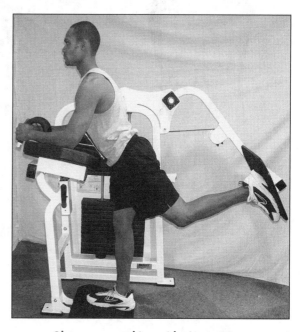

Glute-press machine midpoint position.

In This Chapter

- ◆ Four muscles working together
- ◆ Lunge your way to greatness
- ◆ Learn to bound up stairs
- ◆ Big machines for strong legs

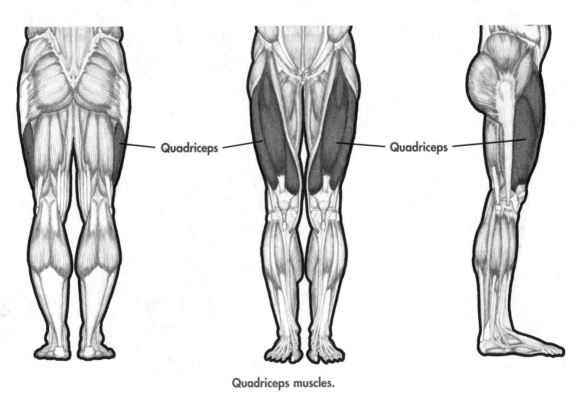

Quadriceps — — Quadriceps

Quadriceps muscles.

Chapter **15**

Become a Thigh Master

Your thighs are the largest muscle group in your lower body and, arguably, the strongest muscle group in your entire body. To become a thigh master, you must know the proper name of the four muscles that make up the quadriceps: the vastus lateralis, vastus medius, vastus intermedius, and rectus femoris (just in case you wanted to learn a little Latin). If you really want to impress your friends, memorize those names so you can tell them exactly what you are working on in the gym.

These muscles often work in partnership with the glutes to help fully extend your leg. The thighs are mainly responsible for straightening your knee, while the glutes straighten your hip. Imagine that you are sitting down (which you probably are right now), and then stand up—you've just used both your thigh and glute muscles in straightening your knee and hip. We focus all our effort in this chapter on the movement of the knee, which brings with it a lot of definition and shape to your knockout legs.

Wall Squat: Level 1

Of the three squat exercises in this chapter, wall squats are the easiest to learn, but they can also be the most difficult to do. Squats are an important part of any knockout workout because the motion itself is so useful in everyday life. On the flip side, the squat has gotten some bad press as being dangerous for your knees. However, if performed correctly, the squat can only improve knee stability. A squat will cause pain or stress to the knees only if it is performed incorrectly, or if you already have knee problems. The wall squat incorporates a stability ball and a wall to provide support until your legs become comfortable with the movement. Try this exercise to determine if deep bending will be okay with your knees.

Preparation

1. Place a stability ball against a wall, and lean against the ball so it is in the curve of your lower back.

2. Place your feet about a foot in front of you, shoulder width apart, with your toes turned slightly out. Put your hands on your hips.

Movement

3. Keep your back and torso as straight as possible while you slowly bend your knees and hips to "squat" until your thighs are parallel with the floor. Now push back up. To really focus on the thighs, think of pushing your feet into the floor—this will concentrate the effort on your quadriceps.

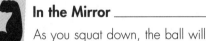

In the Mirror

As you squat down, the ball will roll up toward your shoulders. The ball should never pass your shoulder blades—if it does, start with the ball placed a little lower on your back. Also, as the ball moves up and you move down, concentrate on keeping your back straight; don't let your hips roll back under the ball.

Variations

Level 2: I told you the wall squat could be made more difficult—here's how: use only one leg! Place one foot directly in front of you, and hold the other foot off the ground. Now perform your wall squat using only one leg.

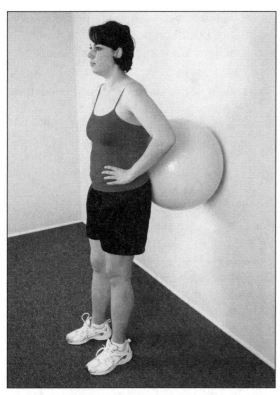

Wall squat beginning and ending position.

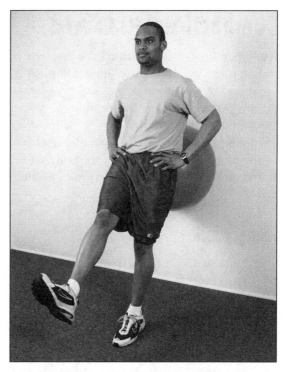

One-leg wall squat beginning and ending position.

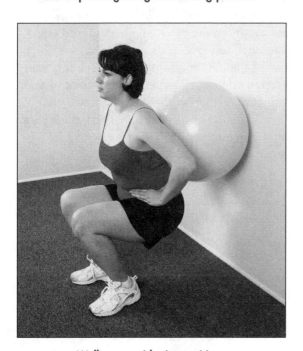

Wall squat midpoint position.

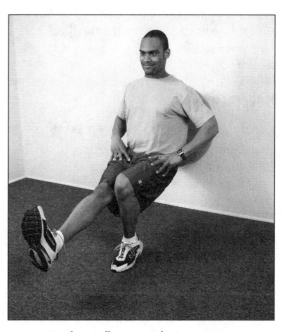

One-leg wall squat midpoint position.

Dumbbell Squat: Level 2

Dumbbell squats really turn up the intensity by adding more weight to your squat. Dumbbell squats mimic the action of picking up objects (in this case heavy objects) off the floor. A good number of back injuries are caused by improper lifting technique in everyday life; dumbbell squats teach you how to keep your body safe and strong while enabling you to still be able to take out the trash.

Preparation

1. Stand with your feet about 4 to 5 inches apart, with your toes slightly turned out.

2. Hold a dumbbell in each hand, with your arms straight and your palms facing your thighs. The dumbbells are there simply to provide more weight—and thus more resistance—so all they have to do is hang. Keep your arms relaxed at your sides during the entire movement (but not so relaxed that you drop the dumbbells on your toes).

Movement

3. Inhale deeply and hold your breath.

4. Bend down as if you are going to set the dumbbells on the ground beside your feet. As you squat, bend both your knees and your hips. Your hips should move out behind you, and your shoulders should lean forward. Really concentrate on keeping your back as straight as possible, and keep your eyes forward (watch yourself in the mirror).

5. Squat until your thighs are parallel to the floor. The dumbbells may or may not touch the floor, depending on how long your arms are.

6. Exhale as you stand back up. Concentrate on pushing your feet into the floor and raising your hips and shoulders at the same time.

Spot Me

The most common mistake you can make with dumbbell squats is to lift your hips and butt in the air first, instead of standing by lifting both the hips and shoulders at the same time. Lifting your hips first places extra stress on your lower back, potentially causing injury.

Variations

Level 3: This exercise can be made to mimic picking up boxes and other objects that you can't hold at your sides like the dumbbells. Instead of holding two dumbbells, hold one dumbbell using both hands (one hand on each end of the dumbbell). Now squat while you keep the dumbbell as close to the front of your body as possible—almost sliding down your legs. When your thighs are parallel, push back up. Remember to keep your back straight.

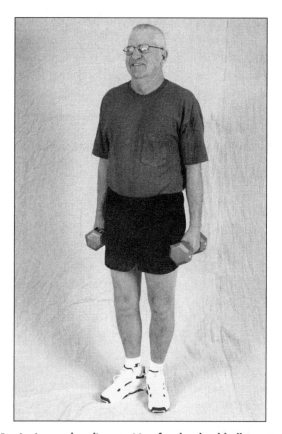

Beginning and ending position for the dumbbell squat.

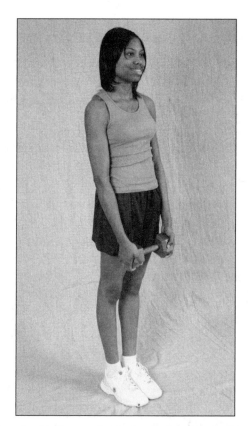

One-dumbbell squat beginning and ending position.

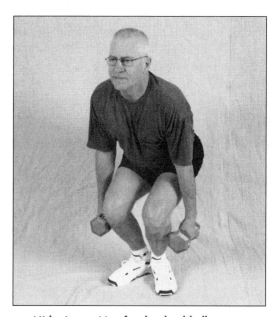

Midpoint position for the dumbbell squat.

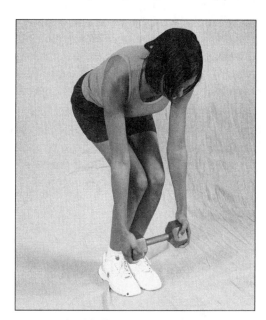

One-dumbbell squat midpoint position.

Leg-Extension Machine: Level 1

The leg-extension machine isolates the quadriceps, helping you create real definition and a knockout look. Almost all leg-extension machines work exactly the same, so this description applies to virtually all manufacturers' machines. This is one exercise that definitely creates a burn in the muscle. This just lets you know that the muscle is working hard—no damage is being done.

Preparation

1. Sit in the machine and adjust the seat back so that your knees line up with the machine's pivot point. This point is always evident (or can be found on the machine's instruction card) and is usually at the edge of the seat. If your knees are too far forward, the beginning part of the exercise will strain your knees.

2. Place your feet behind the footpad. Adjust the height of the pad so that it rests just above your feet, on your shins; you don't want it to push down on the top of your foot. Some machines adjust themselves, so you may not have to do anything here.

3. If the machine has a stack of weights, select your weight; make sure the selector pin is pushed all the way in. If the machine uses plates for resistance, load the plates on the machine before you sit down.

Movement

4. Hold on to the handles and straighten your legs as far as possible. The straighter your legs are, the more benefits you will see.

5. Slowly lower your legs back to the starting position, but don't let the weight stack come to rest. Just before the weights touch, start another rep.

Spot Me

Do this exercise slowly and with control. If you go too fast and "kick" the weight into the air and off your shins, the weight will be impossible to control and could cause injury. Be sure to maintain control and move slowly throughout the exercise.

Variations

Level 2: Most of us have one leg that is stronger than the other, but you can't tell when you work both legs together because the stronger leg helps the weaker leg. As a result, the stronger leg doesn't get enough work itself. To fix this, do this exercise one leg at a time. Just let one leg rest while the other does all the pushing. You may have to use two different weights if there is a big strength deficit in one leg, but the weaker leg will catch up in time.

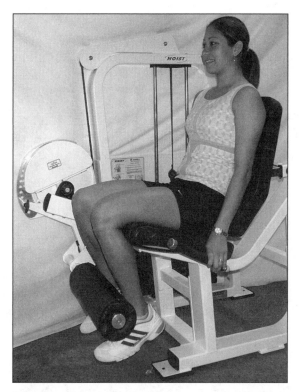

Leg-extension machine beginning and ending position.

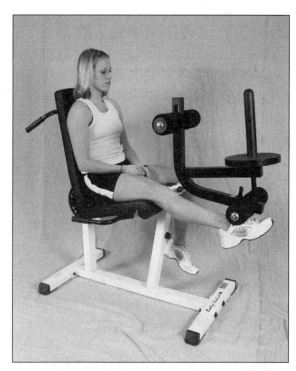

Leg-extension machine, one leg at a time.

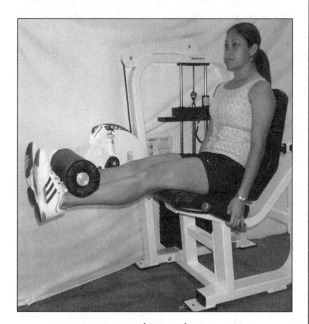

Leg-extension machine midpoint position.

Tubing Extensions: Level 1

If you don't have a gym membership and, therefore, can't get to a leg-extension machine, you can use your resistance tubing to get a similar effect. It's not the same because a machine provides constant resistance: the tubing gets harder the further it stretches. This is a great exercise to take on the road with you because the legs often get ignored during vacation (walking around isn't the same sort of exercise).

Preparation

1. Attach one end of your tubing to something solid at ground level (wrap it around a pole or the foot of a couch or bed).

2. Sit in a chair facing away from the tubing anchor, and slip one foot through the handle of the other end of the tubing. You should start with a little resistance, or stretch, in the tubing when your foot is on the floor directly under your knee. If there is slack in the tubing, scoot your chair farther away until the tubing is tight (extending your leg without any resistance doesn't bring any results).

3. Sit straight in the chair, hold on to the sides of the seat, and extend the leg attached to the tubing in front of you. As your leg extends, the exercise will get harder.

4. Slowly let your leg return to the starting point, and continue repetitions until your set is done. Now do a set on the other leg.

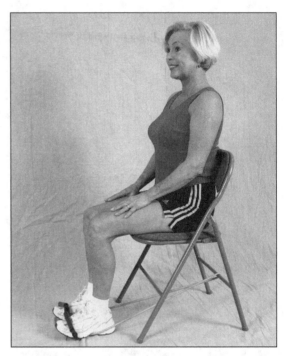

Tubing extension beginning and ending position.

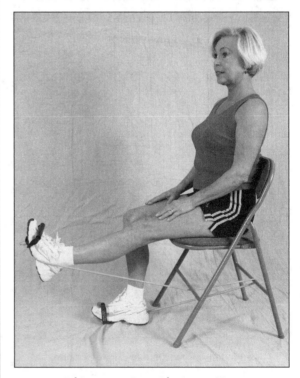

Tubing extension midpoint position.

Variations

Level 2: For more intensity and results, loop the tubing around a pole or something heavy at ground level, and hook one foot into each handle of the tubing. This time you will work both legs at the same time, which causes the tubing to stretch twice as much—providing way more resistance.

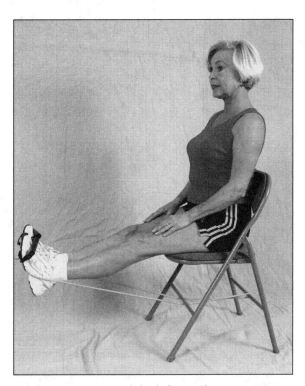

Tubing extension with both feet midpoint position.

Leg Press: Level 1

The leg press is simply a machine version of the squat. With a machine, you can use more resistance under greater control because you don't have to worry about balance, coordination, or keeping your back straight. Several variations of the leg-press machine exist in gyms today, and it's easy to find because it's usually the biggest machine in the room. I prefer the style in which you sit rather than lie down. The sitting position protects your back; the lying position pushes all the weight through your back and shoulders, which is not what we are trying to work on right now.

Preparation

1. Sit in the leg-press machine and place your feet on the platform. Your feet should be spaced slightly wider than shoulder width, with your toes turned out just a bit. Be sure to keep your feet completely on the platform—don't let them hang over the edge.

2. Adjust the seat forward or back until your knees are bent just below 90°. Some machines allow you to adjust the angle of the back rest; this is strictly for your comfort.

3. Select the weight you want to use; make sure the selector pin is pushed all the way in.

Movement

4. Push against the platform with both feet at the same time. When you push, put equal pressure on your heels and the balls of your feet—don't allow the focus to be on your toes, which will make this a calf exercise. Push until your legs are almost completely straight, but don't lock them.

5. Slowly bend your legs, letting the platform move back toward you. When the weights almost touch, start another repetition.

Spot Me

It's nearly impossible to do this exercise wrong, but you can get hurt if you straighten your legs completely and lock your knees at the end. That puts unnecessary pressure on your kneecaps and can strain the joint capsules.

Variations

Level 2: Just as in the leg extension, you can perform this exercise with only one leg to isolate and strengthen one side at a time. Place both feet on the platform in the position described before. Now drop one foot to the floor. This foot placement keeps the working leg pushing straight out. Complete a set with this foot and then switch.

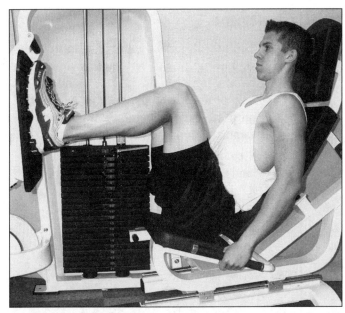

Leg press beginning and ending position.

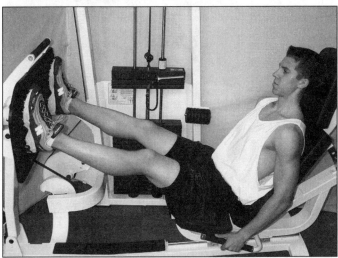

Leg press midpoint position.

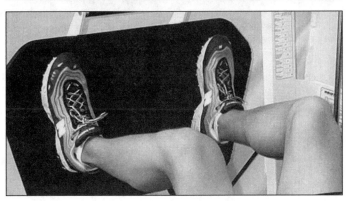

Leg press feet position.

Step-Ups: Level 1

The normal step height on a flight of stairs or sidewalk curb is about 8 inches. That's not very much, which is why stepping up on a curb is not much of an exercise. The step-ups exercise super-sizes the steps you take in everyday life by 200 to 300 percent—more than enough to make those thighs a knockout.

Preparation

1. I recommend a step height of 16 to 24 inches, which is either two or three stair steps. Use any height of step you want—but bigger is better. Choose a height that you'll have to work to get up on but that isn't so high you have to jump back down. You can use a tall stool, an exercise bench, a high-stacked aerobics step, or a flight of stairs.

2. Stand about 6 to 12 inches from the step. If you stand too close, it's harder to get your foot up; if you stand too far away, you must use additional muscles and forward momentum. Place your hands on your hips.

3. Place your right foot on top of the step. Make sure that your foot is completely flat on the step; don't let your heel hang off the edge.

Movement

4. Use the muscles in your right leg to push yourself up. It will be tempting to use your bottom leg (the one on the ground) to help push yourself up, but that defeats the purpose of the exercise. Push until you are standing straight on top of the step.

5. Step down onto your right foot. Try to land toe first, to absorb the impact. The left leg stays on top of the step.

6. Continue the exercise, now pushing up with your left leg. Alternate each leg until you complete the set.

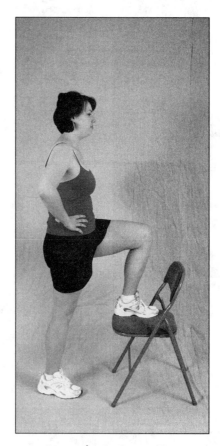

Step-up beginning position.

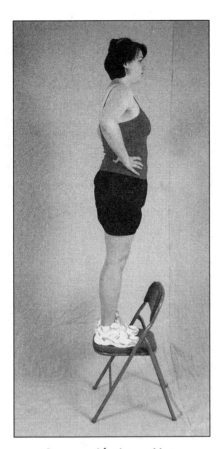

Step-up midpoint position.

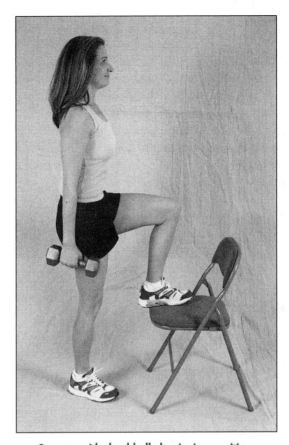

Step-up with dumbbells beginning position.

Variations

Level 2: Add some intensity by holding a dumb-bell in each hand for more resistance. Keep your arms down at your sides for better balance.

Level 3: If you really want to focus on one leg until it's burned out, instead of alternating legs, repeat steps on one side and then do a set on the other side.

Walking Lunges: Level 2

The walking lunge may look slightly clownish, but the results will be nothing to laugh at. Not only will you work the quadriceps, but you'll also work the glutes, which help control the legs and maintain balance. You'll need a long hallway, sidewalk, or track for walking lunges—and remember, however far you go—you have to turn around and come back!

Preparation

1. Start by standing with your hands on your hips, with your feet slightly apart.

Movement

2. Take a giant step forward with one foot. As your foot lands, bend both knees to absorb the impact.

3. Your back knee should move toward the floor but not quite touch it (touching your knee to the floor puts most of your body weight on that one kneecap—not a good idea). When your knee almost touches, push up with the back foot, bringing it forward to meet your front foot. This whole motion resembles stepping over a puddle and getting to the other side.

4. Now step forward with the other foot (so that you alternate working the left and right legs). Continue taking big lunging steps until you've completed your set.

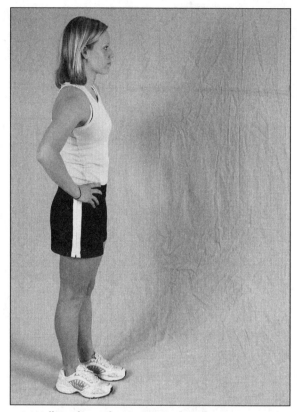

Walking lunge beginning and ending position.

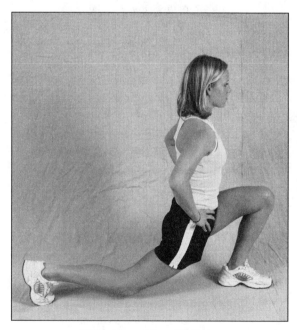

Midpoint position, left foot.

Variations

Level 3: For added intensity, carry a dumbbell in each hand. Let your arms hang by your sides so the dumbbells don't swing.

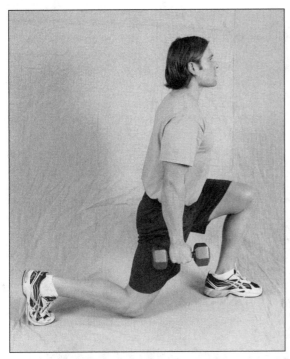

Walking lunge with dumbbells.

Barbell Squat: Level 3

One of the three competitive power-lifting exercises, the barbell squat can be done with huge amounts of weight. (I've actually seen guys with more than 1,000 pounds on the bar.) Fortunately, you won't have to lift anywhere near that amount to get the results you are seeking. Most squat barbells weigh 45 pounds by themselves, which is enough until you become comfortable with the exercise. If this is too much, start with a broomstick. The barbell squat is the most advanced of all the squat exercises, and one of the most difficult exercises in this entire book. With the addition of a bar across your back, safety is a major concern—never do this exercise without a spotter.

Preparation

1. The barbell squat should always be performed inside of a "squat cage." The squat cage has two upright bars that hold the barbell in place while you add weight. With the help of a spotter, add weight to each side of the barbell at the same time (to keep it from tipping over), and use locking collars to secure the weights in place.

2. Adjust the catch bars of the squat cage so that they are just below the level the barbell will reach at full squat. You can determine this level by doing a body squat and noting how low your shoulders get. Place the catch bars just below this point. These bars will allow you to put down the bar and weight without hurting yourself if you ever have trouble completing a repetition.

3. With the barbell resting on the cage, duck under it and position the barbell so that it rests across the top of your shoulders, just below your neck. If the bar feels uncomfortable, wrap it with a towel for extra padding.

4. Stand up with the barbell, take a small step back, and position your feet shoulder width apart, with your toes slightly turned out.

Movement

5. Inhale deeply and hold your breath. Keeping your back as straight as possible, bend your knees and hips simultaneously and begin squatting.

6. As you squat, move your hips behind you and your shoulders forward. Be sure to keep the barbell directly over your feet during the entire movement. Squat until your thighs are parallel with the floor.

7. Exhale and push your feet into the floor as you stand back up. As you stand, be sure to lift your hips and your shoulders at the same time.

Spot Me

Use a spotter and the catch bars! Spotters can help you maintain the correct position and can help you with the weight when you get tired. The catch bars are even more important than the spotter—they prevent the bar from squishing you into the floor if you can't finish a repetition.

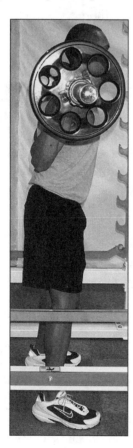
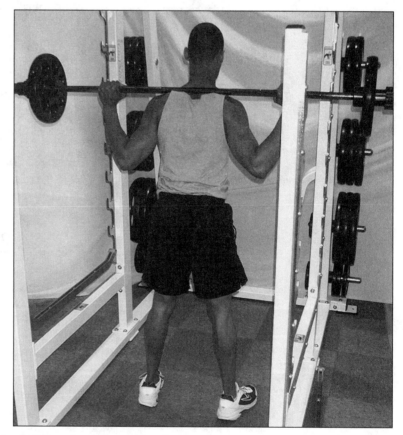

Barbell squat beginning and ending position.

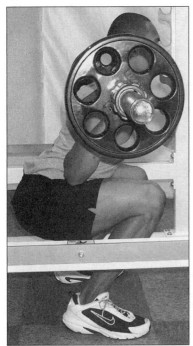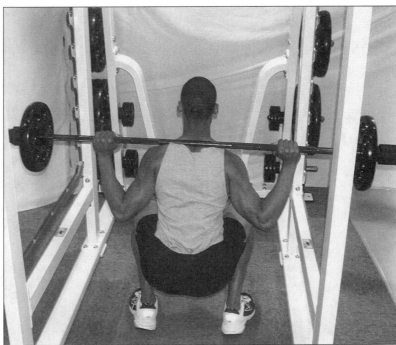

Barbell squat midpoint position.

In This Chapter

◆ Long, skinny muscles

◆ One muscle, three machines

◆ Building a muscle bridge

◆ The opposite of extension

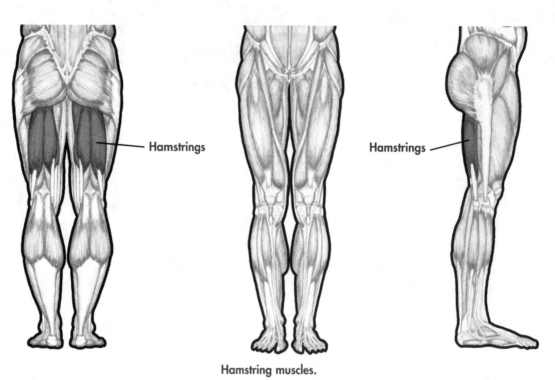

Hamstrings

Hamstrings

Hamstring muscles.

Chapter 16

Tug on Your Hamstrings

Reach around and grab the back of your leg just below your butt. You are holding the hamstring muscles. Most muscle groups in your body are named for what they do or how they are designed—all except for the hamstrings. This muscle group is made up of three different muscles: the semitendonosus, semimembranosus, and biceps femoris. So why are they called hamstrings? From what I have been able to discover, butchers used to hang the ham portion of a pig by the tendons of these muscles; since these tendons were long and skinny, they resembled strings—therefore, "ham-strings" or hamstrings.

How does this affect you? It doesn't. It's just a neat bit of trivia you can hold on to. What does affect you is the way these muscles are used. Without them, you would walk like Frankenstein's monster because your knees couldn't bend. That's why what the hamstrings do—bend your knees—is called flexion. Everyday activities such as walking, running, and climbing stairs, would be almost impossible without knee flexion.

It's hard to see your hamstrings in the mirror, but as with your back muscles, people behind and to the side of you will notice them. Knockout hamstrings give the back of your leg a great shape to balance the look of your knockout thighs. These muscles are most obvious when the legs are slightly bent at the knees—that's where these muscles are contracting the most. But whatever position you are in, knockout hamstrings will add to the contours of your backside and make your legs stand out in a crowd.

Lying Machine Curls: Level 1

The lying leg-curl machine is the oldest of all the hamstring exercises. This style of machine has been around as long as anyone can remember. The position may be a bit awkward to get into and out of, and not all machines are built the same way. Some of them have a flat bench to lay on, some have a bench that is bent upward near your hips for more comfort, and some have special pads for your elbows and arms. Whatever model of machine you are using, this exercise is always highly effective.

Preparation

1. Determine the location of the knee pivot point on the machine. Most of the time, lying leg-curl machines are designed so that the pivot point is right at the edge of the padding. If this is what you see, stand at the end of the bench with your knees right against the padding, and lie down. Your kneecaps should hang off the end of the bench.

2. Some machines have pads for your elbows to rest on; others have a flat bench with handles underneath to hang on to. Either way, lie down flat and put your elbows and hands in the proper position.

3. Your Achilles tendon (just above your heel) should be underneath the leg pad. Some machines adjust this pad automatically, but if not, adjust it so that it is not pushing down on your heel or foot.

4. Select the weight you want to use; make sure the selector pin is pushed all the way in. If your machine uses plates for resistance, add the weight before you lie down.

Movement

5. Bend your knees and try to bring the foot pad all the way up to touch your butt. The farther you can "curl" your legs, the more you get out of the exercise.

6. Slowly let the bar back down until the weights almost touch; then start another rep.

In the Mirror

As the weights increase and the intensity rises, your hips will want to lift as you curl with your legs. This is a normal body reaction to the mechanics of the exercise, but it decreases the effectiveness of the exercise. You can prevent this and focus on the hamstrings by pushing your hips into the pad as you are curling your legs.

Variations

Level 2: Since one leg will almost always be stronger than the other in the beginning, you can focus your exercise on each leg individually to make them more balanced and increase the intensity of the exercise. Lie in the same position, and just let one leg rest while the other leg does all the curling.

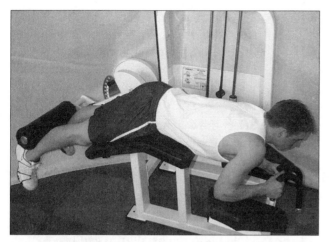

Lying machine curl beginning and ending position.

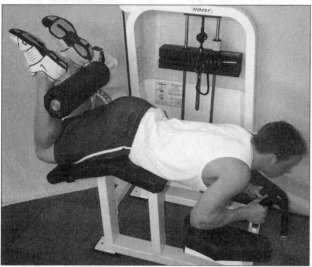

Lying machine curl midpoint position.

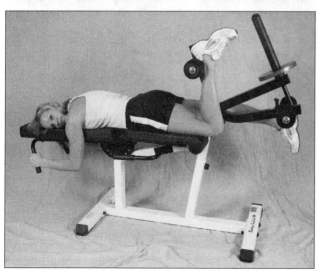

Lying machine curl using only one leg.

Seated Machine Curls: Level 1

Seated leg-curl machines came on the market a few years ago and have quickly become more popular than the lying-down design. Just like the lying machine curl, they target and isolate the hamstring muscles. A benefit of the seated leg-curl machine is that it's easier to get into and out of, and you won't have to lie facedown on a bench to do it. The downside to the seated leg-curl machine is that it offers a decreased range of motion compared to the lying leg-curl machine—so it takes more work to get the same knockout results.

Preparation

1. Sit on the machine and adjust the seat back so that your knees line up with the machine's pivot point. The seat is usually quite short on these machines and may stop about halfway to your knees, so be sure to identify the proper pivot point.

2. Put your feet and legs on top of the leg pad. You may have to adjust the leg pad so that it is in contact with your Achilles tendon and is not pushing on your foot.

3. Use the thigh pad to hold yourself in the seat—otherwise, when you push down on the leg pad, your knees will rise up and nothing will happen. Adjust the thigh pad until it's just snug against the top of your legs.

4. Select the weight you want to use; make sure the selector pin is pushed all the way in.

Movement

5. Hold on to the hand grips and bend your knees, pulling the leg pad down and under the seat. Pretend you are trying to kick yourself in the butt—although the machine will stop you before you do.

6. At the end of your pull, give it an extra little squeeze to get a little bit farther—every inch counts.

7. Slowly straighten your legs until the weights almost touch; then start another repetition.

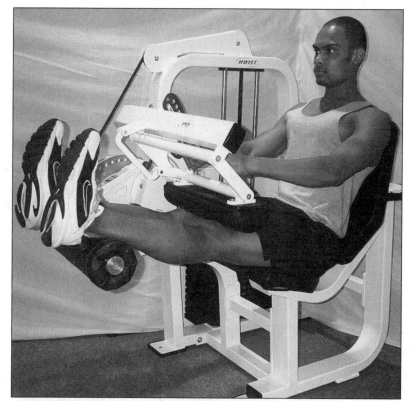

Seated machine curl beginning and ending position.

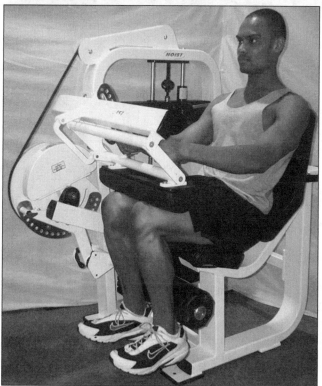

Seated machine curl midpoint position.

Standing Curl: Level 2

The standing curl is perhaps the most relevant hamstring machine to everyday life. It's pretty rare that we are lying down or seated and have to bend our knees against any sort of resistance. Most of the time, we are standing up when our hamstrings are working (walking, climbing stairs, and so on), so it makes sense to work them in a standing position. This is a more advanced exercise because you have to balance on one leg while the other leg is working, and you have to keep your body straight the whole time. You won't be able to use as much weight on this exercise because only one leg will be working, but the effects will definitely be worth the effort.

Preparation

1. Stand in the machine facing the weight stack. Other than the thigh pad that allows you to choose either the right or the left leg, there usually isn't anything to adjust other than the amount of weight you are using. Pick which leg you want to work and flip the thigh pad to that side.

2. Hold on to the handles and stand as straight as possible. The effort of this exercise makes you want to lean forward in an attempt to get the weight all the way up—don't. Stay straight and tall.

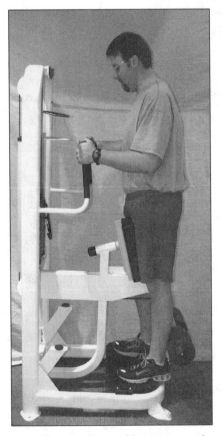

Standing machine curl beginning and ending position.

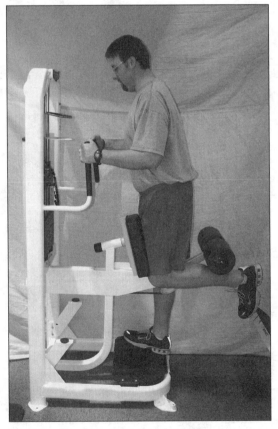

Standing machine curl midpoint position for left leg.

Movement

3. Slowly bend one knee and lift the heel pad up as far as you can—all the way to your butt, if possible.

4. Let the pad down slowly, allowing the muscles to work on the way down. Repeat until your set is complete; then flip the thigh pad to the other side and work that leg.

Variations

Level 1: If you don't have a machine, you can still do this exercise with ankle weights. Strap ankle weights on your legs, stand facing a wall, and perform the leg curl with one leg and then the other, alternating left and right curls.

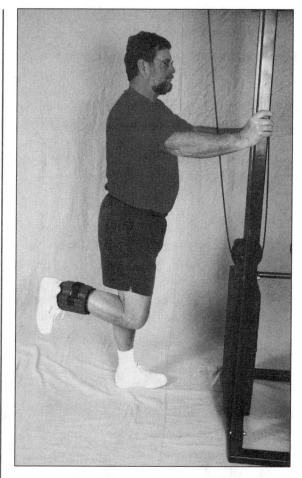

Standing curl with ankle weight.

Tubing Pulls: Level 1

Resistance tubing is a great tool to use with the hamstrings—especially while traveling. Just like all tubing exercises, this one will get harder the farther you stretch out that tubing—but that just means the results will be even better. You can use this exercise to isolate one leg at a time or work both legs together. Either way, it's simple and effective.

Preparation

1. Attach one end of your resistance tubing to a pole, a machine, or something really heavy at ground level.

2. Slide the toe of one foot through the other handle and wrap the tubing around your shin a couple times to keep it in place. If you don't wrap the tubing around your shin, it will slip off halfway through the exercise. It helps if you are wearing socks so the tubing doesn't rub against your skin.

3. Sit in a chair facing the anchor with your leg straight out in front of you. Move the chair back until the tubing has a little stretch to it.

Movement

4. Keep your other foot on the floor, keep your hands holding on to the chair sides, and pull your foot toward you and under the chair as far as possible.

5. Slowly let your foot back out and start another repetition. Finish that set and switch legs.

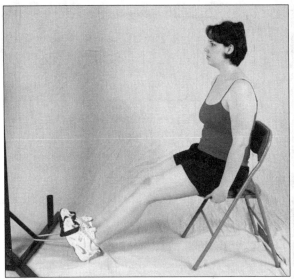

Tubing pull beginning and ending position.

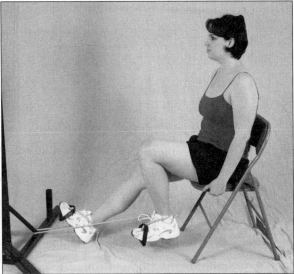

Tubing pull midpoint position.

Variations

Level 2: Work both legs at the same time by looping the tubing around a pole at ground level and hooking one foot into each of the handles. Loop the tubing around each shin to keep it in place. Now start with both legs in front of you, and pull them both back under the chair.

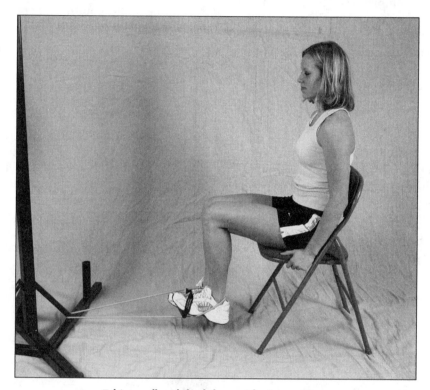

Tubing pull with both legs midpoint position.

Lying Bridges: Level 2

A little-known thing about the hamstrings is that they not only bend the knees, but they also help straighten the hips. Usually we concentrate on the glutes to straighten the hips, but the hamstrings can be emphasized at the hip joint and worked in a whole new way. This exercise may seem pretty simple to begin with, but after you give it a set or two, you'll understand what I mean when I say it will give your hamstrings a burn like no other exercise can.

Preparation

1. Lie on your back on a carpeted surface or an exercise mat. Bend your knees and keep your feet flat on the floor. Your heels should be about 18 inches away from your butt.
2. Place both hands at your sides, with your palms pressing down against the floor.

Movement

3. In one smooth motion, lift your hips until your knees, hips, and shoulders are in a straight line. Do not lift your hips to the point that you can't see your knees. You can push against the floor with your hands to help lift your hips if you need to, but try not to.
4. Slowly relax and lower your hips back to the ground.

Spot Me

Since you are supporting a lot of weight on the top of your shoulders and the base of your neck, you might feel some strain in these areas. If so, immediately relax and rest before you attempt another repetition. If you experience any pain in your neck from this exercise, stop and consult with your doctor before you attempt it again.

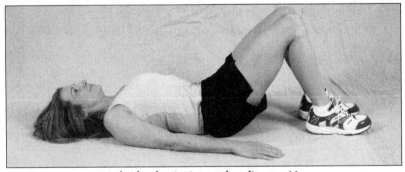

Lying bridge beginning and ending position.

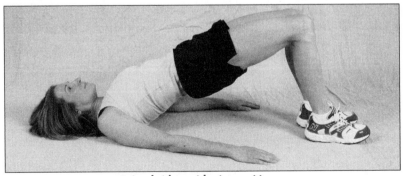

Lying bridge midpoint position.

Variations

Level 3: Double the intensity by making only one leg lift the weight of your body off the floor. Hold one leg straight out in the air while the other leg does all the work.

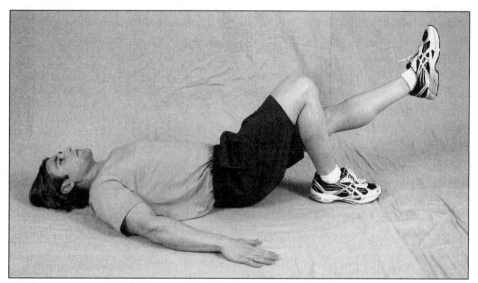

Lying bridge one leg beginning and ending position.

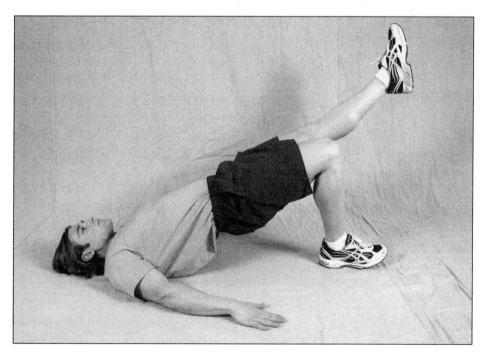

Lying bridge one leg midpoint position.

Lean Forward: Level 3

This last exercise for the hamstrings is so hard that I've seen only a handful of people be able to complete this exercise through its full range of motion. However, the neat thing about this exercise is that you don't have to complete the full range of motion to get the most benefits. In fact, you may actually move less during this exercise than any other exercise (including crunches). The secret to the effectiveness of this move is the weight of your body. That's not exactly a secret, but it is the key. Your body weight acts as the resistance, and because of physics and gravity, the leverage your body weight has during this move is tremendous—as are the results of doing it.

Preparation

1. Kneel on the ground with your feet anchored under a heavy object like a machine, or with a partner holding them down for you.

2. Keep your body straight from the knees to the shoulders. Hold your hands in front of you to help catch yourself, if necessary.

Movement

3. Slowly lean your entire body forward until you start to feel your hamstrings tighten. They are trying to keep you from falling forward, so they'll be working immediately.

4. Lean out as far as you can without falling; then pull yourself back using those same muscles. Now is when you will feel them working their hardest.

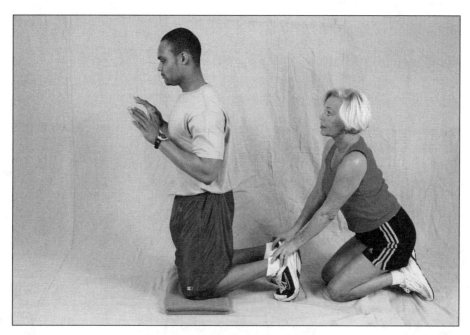

Lean forward beginning and ending position.

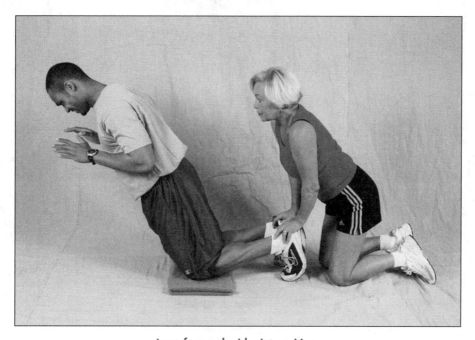

Lean forward midpoint position.

In This Chapter

- ◆ The reason for high heels
- ◆ Getting up on your tippy-toes
- ◆ If there's a step, you can exercise
- ◆ Powering your endurance exercise

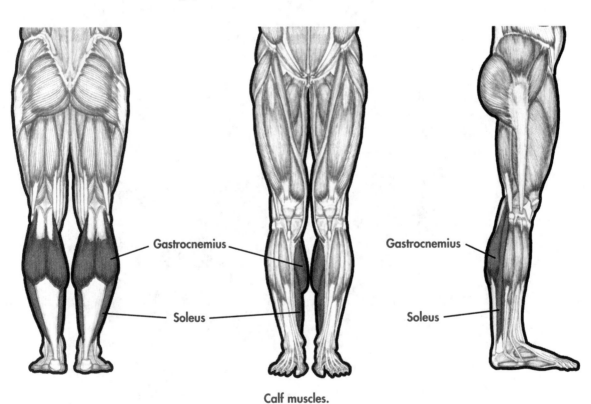

Calf muscles.

Chapter 17

The First Muscles Above Your Feet

Did you know that high-heel shoes were invented for women to help define the calf muscles? It's true! When you push yourself up onto your toes, the calf muscles contract. If you keep the leg in that position, you show off the calves all the time. The calves are also one of the most important muscle groups for walking and running. Try to walk without pushing off with your toes—it's that Frankenstein thing all over again. These muscles work all the time—every time you walk, run, or try to make yourself look taller.

Every one of the muscles that control your feet, toes, and ankles is contained in the calves (thank goodness for that—otherwise you'd have muscle-bound feet). We aren't concerned with working your ankles, feet, and toes because they get plenty of work while you walk around all day, but we do need to focus a little on the two strong muscles in your calves—the gastrocnemius and soleus. These two muscles give your calves a distinct muscular definition that really puts the finishing touch on a set of knockout legs.

Calf-Raise Machine: Level 1

Old-style calf-raise machines made you stand under a couple of shoulder pads and hold the weight on your shoulders and back. Those machines ended up hurting people's shoulders more than they helped their calves, so a new style of calf-raise machine has evolved. This new machine lets you sit and absorb the weight through your hips. These are sometimes called angled calf machines or 45° calf-raise machines. But whatever it's called, this machine isolates the calves and can push you beyond what you thought your calves could look like.

Preparation

1. The calf-raise machine has a pivot point around which the footplate moves. Using the instruction card on the machine, identify this point. Place your feet on the footplace, letting your heels hang off the bottom edge so they line up with this pivot point. In most cases, only the balls of your feet and your toes will actually be on the footplate.

2. Adjust the seat so that your legs are almost completely straight, but not totally. You want them to still have a little bit of bend in them.

3. Select the weight that you want to use, making sure the selector pin is pushed all the way in.

Movement

4. Push out on the footplate with the balls of your feet. The goal is to push your toes as far away from you as you can, getting the calf muscles to completely flex.

5. Slowly let the toes move back toward you, relaxing the calves.

In the Mirror

About the only way you can do this exercise wrong is to turn it into a leg press. This happens if your seat is placed too close and your knees are too bent. If you see your knees moving during this exercise, you've turned it into a leg press. Be sure to move the seat back to make the most of your calf workout.

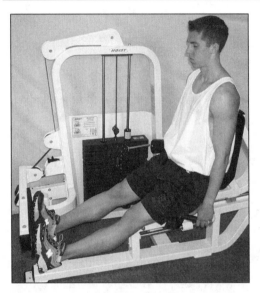

Calf-raise machine beginning and ending position.

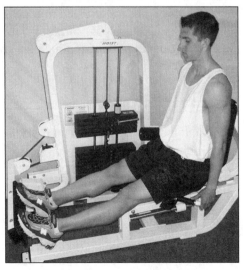

Calf-raise machine midpoint position.

Seated Calf Raise: Level 1

The seated calf raise targets and isolates the soleus muscle in the calf. The soleus muscle is mainly an endurance muscle that's worked when you go for long walks, ride your bike, or climb stairs. Making it stronger will allow you to do more fat-burning cardio work. Because it's located under the gastrocnemius muscle, the soleus muscle is generally not as visible, so you won't see as much flexing—but don't let that fool you. Developing the soleus muscle will have a direct impact on endurance activities, helping you reach your knockout workout goals on two fronts.

Preparation

1. Place the weight you want to use on the machine.

2. Sit in the seat, place your feet on the footplate, and slide your knees under the knee pads. Only your toes and the balls of your feet should be on the footplate; the rest of your foot should hang out over the edge. Adjust the knee pads so that they are snug against your knees—any space between your knees and the knee pad prevents you from doing this exercise correctly.

3. Most machines have handgrips on top of the knee pads for you to hang on to. You can hold on to these, or you can put your hands in your lap. If you do hold on to the handles, make sure you don't "pull" the knee pad up using your arms instead of your calf muscles.

Movement

4. Push on the balls of your feet to raise your heels as high as possible. On the first repetition, the bar that supports the machine and weight will move out of the way.

5. Lower your heels as far as you can to the "down" position. When you can't stretch the calf any further, push up on the balls of your feet again. Raise your heels as far as you can to get to the "up" position.

6. Repeat lowering and raising your heels for a full set. On the last repetition, when your heels are at the highest point, move the bar that supports the machine and weight back into place, and slowly lower your heels back to the starting point.

Spot Me

Don't try to get out of the machine until the support bar is back in place. The support bar holds the extra weight you added. If you try to slide your knees out of the machine without using the support bar, you may injure your legs or damage the machine.

Variations

Level 1: You can do this exercise even if you don't have a special machine. Sit on the edge of a bench or chair. The bench's height should allow your thighs to rest parallel to the floor. A bench that's too high or too low decreases the impact of this exercise. Sit with your feet together, flat on the floor. For resistance, place a weight plate or dumbbell on your knees. Now push up on the balls of your feet as high as you can. If you can make it up to the tips of your toes, you'll get even more out of this exercise.

Level 2: Increase the intensity of this calf exercise by working one leg at a time. Straighten one leg in front of you and let it rest while exercising the other calf.

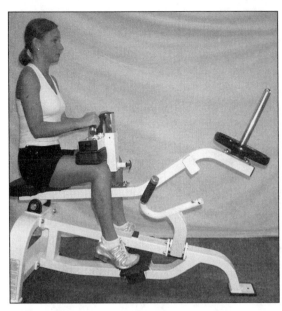

Seated calf raise beginning and ending position.

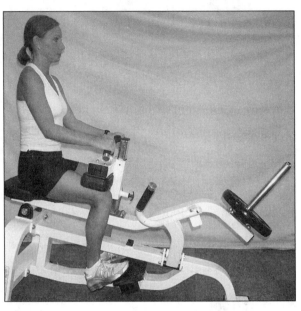

Seated calf raise midpoint position.

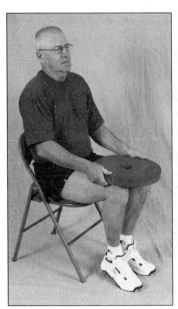

Seated calf raise without a machine beginning and ending position.

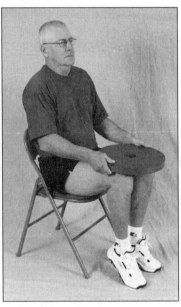

Seated calf raise without a machine midpoint position.

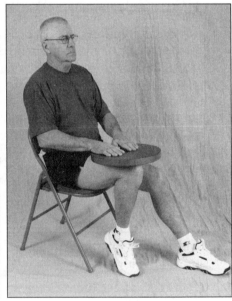

One-leg version of the seated calf raise.

Toe Press: Level 1

This exercise uses your body weight and the pressure you create against a wall for resistance. The toe press is pretty cool because you can do it anywhere—without machines or equipment—and you can make it more intense by adjusting your body position and the pressure you create. You can actually double the resistance created by your body weight by pushing against the wall in some cases—which is usually more than enough to create knockout calves.

Preparation

1. Stand about an arm's length away from a wall. Place both hands against the wall for support and balance.
2. Keep your feet together and flat on the floor.

Movement

3. Push up on the balls of your feet to make yourself as tall as possible (up on your tippy toes, if you can).
4. Slowly lower yourself back down and repeat reps until you have finished your set.

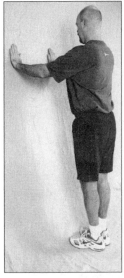 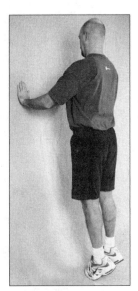

Toe press beginning and ending position.   Toe press midpoint position.

Variations

Level 2: To make this exercise more intense, add resistance by moving your feet farther away from the wall and pushing against the wall with your hands. The farther your feet are from the wall and the harder you push against the wall, the more your calves will have to work to lift you up.

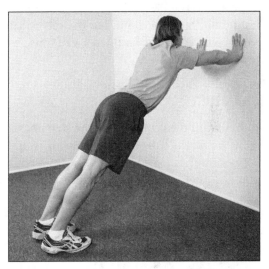

Toe press level 2 beginning and ending position.

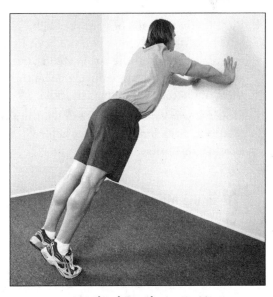

Toe press level 2 midpoint position.

Stair Press: Level 1

You can do the stair press anywhere there is a flight of stairs, a curb, an aerobics bench, or something similar—which is just about everywhere. Stair presses are the most basic of all calf exercises. They are a staple of most people's leg workouts because they provide a great deal of definition by working both the gastrocnemius and the soleus muscles. This movement provides the full range of motion of the calves, and the full involvement of both large calf muscles together.

Preparation

1. Stand on the very edge of the step or curb with just the balls of your feet and your toes on the step.
2. Let your heels drop toward the floor as far as possible.
3. Hold on to the wall or another object to keep your balance.

Movement

4. Push up on the balls of your feet as high as possible. Make sure that you use both legs and really get up in the air. Pretend you are trying to reach something on the top shelf, and stretch as high as possible.
5. Slowly lower your heels back down toward the floor, stretching the calves before another repetition.

In the Mirror

As you rise up and down, your feet will work themselves off the edge of the bench. Stop occasionally and reposition your feet.

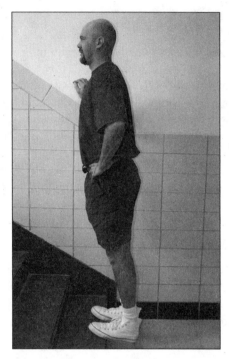

Stair press beginning and ending position.

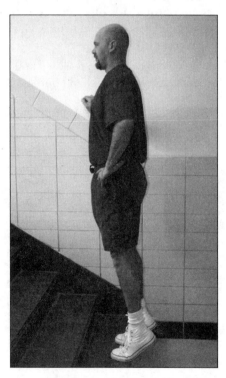

Stair press midpoint position.

Variations

Level 2: For a really intense version of this exercise, use only one leg at a time. Crossing one foot behind the other puts all your body weight on one leg, making the calf muscles work twice as hard.

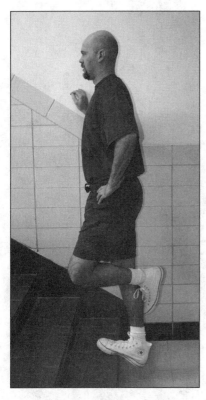

Stair press with one foot.

Glossary

aerobic class   Group exercise in which participants follow an instructor as they perform rhythmic movements along with exercise. Forms of aerobic classes include step aerobics, pump aerobics, and cardio-kickboxing aerobics.

aerobic exercise   Exercises that increase your heart rate and focus on improving the fitness of your heart muscle. Also known as cardiovascular exercise.

apple shape   A body shape defined by a large chest, increased abdominal and stomach fat, and a narrow waist and hips.

balance   The ability to move though exercise and daily movements without falling down.

basal metabolic rate (BMR)   The number of calories required to keep you alive at rest, without any movement. The average BMR is 1,200 to 2,000 calories a day.

bodybuilding   A form of exercise that focuses on developing as much muscle mass and size as possible.

body-fat percentage   The amount of your body that is made up of fat, calculated as a percentage of your entire body weight.

body type   A very general description of the body based on the size of your muscles and the distribution of fat. There are three basic body types: mesomorph, ectomorph, and endomorph. *See also* specific listings.

calorie A unit of energy. The amount of heat needed to raise the temperature of 1 gram of water 1°. Also used as a measure of the amount of energy contained in food.

carbohydrate A nutrient that provides 4 calories in every gram. The main source of energy for high-intensity exercise and for the brain and nervous system.

cardiovascular exercise *See* aerobic exercise.

circular progression A method of progression that is based on the particular repetition range for each workout goal and that allows you to continually see improvements.

complex carbohydrate A category of carbohydrates also called starches. Examples are grains, cereals, vegetables, and dried beans and peas.

cookie-cutter plan A very basic workout that you normally find in fitness magazines. Designed for the general population, but not individualized for anyone's particular goals.

cool-down A short period of time at the end of aerobic exercise when the intensity is lowered to allow the heart rate to return to its resting level.

coordination The ability to move your body in smooth and fluid motions, and to complete exercise skills with ease.

definition A characteristic of muscle that allows you to "see" the shape of the muscle, usually by increasing the muscle's mass or decreasing the layer of fat that typically covers a muscle and hides it.

dehydration A condition in which the body is low on water. Symptoms include dry mouth, thirst, and lack of sweat. If serious, it can lead to heat exhaustion and heat stroke.

ectomorph A body type characterized by a tall, slender build with very little fat or muscle definition.

endomorph A body type characterized by a short, heavy, rounded build with extra body fat and a lack of muscle definition.

exercise physiology The study of how exercise affects the body.

exercise prescription (ExRx) Terminology used by fitness and medical professionals for an exercise program.

fad diet A diet that typically restricts calories, exempts certain foods, or allows you to eat only certain foods. Fad diets usually are not a nutritional option and can rarely be continued for more than a few weeks without disrupting key body systems.

fat A nutrient that provides 9 calories in every gram. Essential in the diet, yet often consumed in excess, leading to stores of fat in the body.

Food Guide Pyramid A nutrition program based on sound scientific research, and designed by hundreds of nutrition experts along with the U.S. government. The Food Guide Pyramid divides foods into groups and provides guidelines on the amount and type of foods that should be consumed from each group.

full-body workout A workout program that includes exercises for every muscle group in your body during one session.

game plan A system to make sure you are using the right exercises for your body. This is your individual workout design based on your goals and needs. Includes exercises, sets, and repetitions. *See also* set, repetition.

genetics Your DNA sequence inherited from your parents that determines your basic bone shape, your chances of developing certain diseases, and your facial characteristics.

gravity A force of nature that pulls down on everything. The force of gravity determines your weight and the weight of all objects. If you weigh 100 pounds, that means there is 100 pounds of gravitational force pushing down on you.

heart disease   Any number of heart-related illnesses, including coronary heart disease, atherosclerosis, and congestive heart failure.

heart-rate monitor   A device that measures your heart rate while you are working out. Typically consists of a strap worn across the chest to transmit your heart rate to a watch worn on your wrist.

heart-rate training zone   The heart-rate range that allows you to make the most improvement in the fitness of your heart muscle.

hitting the wall   A term that fitness enthusiasts use to describe the sensation of running out of carbs for energy. It feels like you actually ran into a wall: your body slows down, you have trouble thinking straight, and there is no way you can go on until you refuel. The only way to avoid this is to keep your body fed with carbohydrates.

indoor aerobic machine   Any piece of equipment designed to increase your heart rate for aerobic exercise. Examples include treadmills, bikes, and stair-climbers.

intensity   A measure of how hard you are working, usually related to aerobic exercise.

inversely proportional   Characterized by having opposite effects. As one goes up, the other goes down.

Jazzercise   An early form of aerobic classes made popular by the combination of jazz dance moves and rhythmic movements to music.

journaling   Keeping track of your workouts in a notebook so that you can look back to see what has worked for you and to note your progress.

knockout   Term used to describe anything that is sensationally striking, appealing, or attractive.

knockout workout   An exercise program designed to give your body a knockout look.

maintenance program   A workout that does not progress, but that stays the same so that you will not lose any of the progress you already made—similar to a routine.

maximum heart rate   The fastest your heart can possibly beat, mainly determined by your age. Estimated by using the formula 220 – age.

meal replacement   Supplements that contain a large number of calories and are marketed as food that can be consumed in place of a regular meal.

mesomorph   A body type characterized by a good amount of muscle and a small amount of fat. Typically medium height and muscular build.

metabolism   The number of calories your body burns just to keep your primary functions (heartbeat, respiration, blood flow) working. Metabolism is measured as the number of calories you burn during a 24-hour period while lying still.

muscle mass   The amount of muscle distributed in any one area. One goal of a knockout workout is to increase muscle mass.

nutrient   Food that provides energy. Only carbohydrates, protein, and fat are nutrients.

nutritionist   Any person who knows what a food is can claim to be a nutritionist. This is not a nutrition expert.

one-size-fits-all exercise plan   General exercise plans typically seen in fitness magazines that are not designed for anyone in particular, and that usually will not work as advertised because of individual differences.

pear shape   A body shape characterized by wide hips and extra fat accumulation below the waist, combined with narrow shoulders and chest.

perceived exertion   How hard you feel you are working.

personal trainer An individual who has studied exercise physiology and is certified to design exercise programs.

plateau A period of time during which you have stopped getting any results from your workout.

progression Consistently intensifying your workout so that it remains a challenge and brings continual improvements.

protein A nutrient that provides 4 calories in every gram. Essential for building muscle and controlling the body systems.

pulse Your heart rate as measured at your wrist or on your neck.

rating of perceived exertion (RPE) A numeric way of describing how you feel you are working as a whole, including how hard your muscles are working, how hard you are breathing, and how tired you feel.

registered dietician (RD) A person who has earned a college degree in nutrition and is certified by the American Dietetics Association.

repetition Typically considered the lifting and lowering of a weight one time, or one full exercise movement. A number of repetitions make up an exercise set. *See also* set.

resistance The object or force that pushes back against you and tries to prevent you from moving. In the case of a knockout workout, the resistance can be the weight of the dumbbell, barbell, or the setting on a cardiovascular machine.

resistance tubing A long piece of rubber tubing, about 3 feet long, with handles on each end. It can be used as resistance instead of using barbells or dumbbells.

resting heart rate How fast your heart beats while you are at rest.

routine An exercise program that does not change, meaning that you will not get any further results from the program.

set A number of repetitions completed together. A set can contain anywhere from 1 to 16 repetitions. *See also* repetition.

split workout A workout that is divided into two or more parts so that the entire workout is not completed in one session. A split workout can be divided into separate sessions on the same day or over two consecutive days.

stability ball A large ball filled with air that can be used as a chair or exercise bench.

supplement Foods that should be used in addition to regular foods to increase the number of calories consumed or to provide vitamins and minerals missing from the diet.

weight training Any exercise that uses an external form of resistance such as a barbell or exercise machine.

Resources

Exercise Equipment

Fitness First
P.O. Box 251
Shawnee Mission, KS 66201
1-800-421-1791
www.fitness1st.com

M-F Athletic/Perform Better
11 Amflex Dr.
Cranston, RI 02920
1-800-682-6950
www.performbetter.com

Power Systems
P.O. Box 31709
Knoxville, TN 37930
1-800-321-6975
www.power-systems.com

Sportsmith
5925 S. 118th East Ave.
Tulsa, OK 74146
1-800-713-2880
www.sportsmith.net

SPRI Products, Inc.
1600 Northwind Blvd.
Libertyville, IL 60048
1-800-222-7774
www.spriproducts.com

Personal Trainers

American College of Sports Medicine
P.O. Box 1440
Indianapolis, IN 46206
1-800-486-5643
www.acsm.org

IDEA Health and Fitness Association
10455 Pacific Center Ct.
San Diego, CA 92121
1-800-999-IDEA
www.ideafit.com

National Strength and Conditioning
Association
1885 Bob Johnson Dr.
Colorado Springs, CO 80906
1-800-815-6826
www.nsca.com

Nutrition Info

U.S. Department of Agriculture—Consumer
Corner
Official site of Food, Nutrition, and Consumer
Services
www.nal.usda.gov/fnic/consumersite/allabout-
food.htm

U.S. Food and Drug Administration (FDA)
5600 Fishers Lane
Rockville, MD 20857
1-888-463-6332
www.fda.gov

American Dietetic Association
120 S. Riverside Plaza, Suite 2000
Chicago, IL 60606-6995
1-800-877-1600
www.eatright.org

Nutrition Analysis and Tools
(Sponsored by the University of Illinois;
includes a nutrition-analysis tool, an energy cal-
culator, and links to other nutrition sites)
http://nat.crgq.com

Food Guide Pyramid
United States Department of Agriculture
www.mypyramid.gov or www.mypyramid.com

Other Good Books

Bauer, Joy, RD. *The Complete Idiot's Guide to Total Nutrition.* Indianapolis: Alpha Books, 2005.

Hagerman, Patrick S., Ed.D. *The Complete Idiot's Guide to Core Conditioning Illustrated.* Indianapolis: Alpha Books, 2006.

Hagerman, Patrick S., Ed.D., with Randall Broderdorf and Jennifer Lata Rung. *The Complete Idiot's Guide to Body Sculpting Illustrated.* Indianapolis: Alpha Books, 2004.

Weatherwax, Dawn. *The Complete Idiot's Guide to Sports Nutrition.* Indianapolis: Alpha Books, 2003.

Index

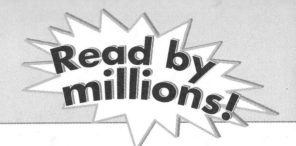
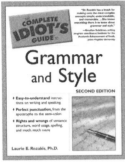
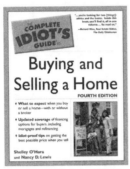
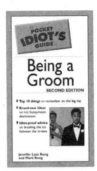
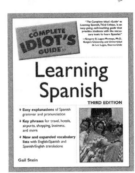
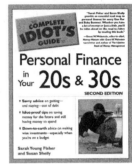
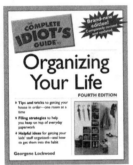
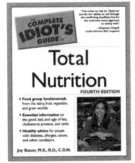
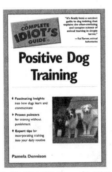
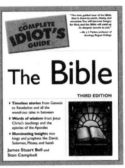
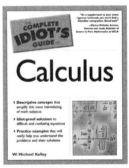
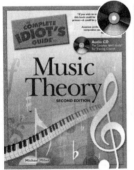
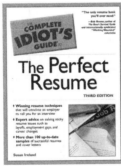
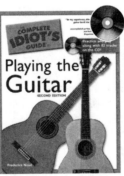
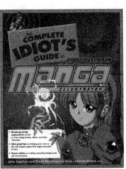
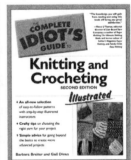